PRAISE

Mirth is God's Medicine

"Told from the unique perspective of an internist, someone keenly familiar with the ins and outs of the medical system, Dr. Heather Thompson provides a glimpse into the therapeutic process, seen through the fresh eyes of a vulnerable patient. From her vantage point, she soon realizes that we are all connected, and that the medical journey of one woman's breast cancer diagnosis, treatment, and care involves a whole host of individuals from the radiologist who reads the scans to the scheduler who facilitates appointments."

—Margaret Lesh, Author of *Let Me Get This Off My Chest: A Breast Cancer Survivor Over-Shares*

"Every woman's journey through breast cancer is different, driven by the biology and stage of disease as well as personal treatment preferences. But, all share the common experience of dealing with the possibility, and then the reality, of a potentially life threatening diagnosis. In *Mirth is God's Medicine*, Heather Thompson provides us with a frank, often humorous account of the experience of a physician navigating a breast cancer diagnosis and treatment. The variety of coping strategies and support systems she employs offer something for all patients and their families. For medical professionals, this candid description of a self described evidence based practitioner's thought processes and reactions to diagnosis and treatment provides valuable insights into why purely fact based discussions about treatment don't always achieve the desired results, and reminds us that regardless of background and education, a new breast cancer diagnosis is often overwhelming."

—Monica Morrow, MD, Chief of Breast Surgery at Memorial Sloan Kettering Cancer Center in Manhattan, New York and author of *Managing Breast Cancer Risk, Diseases of the Breast, and Breast Cancer for Dummies*

PRAISE

Mirth is God's Medicine

"For anyone who has dealt with, or is in the process of dealing with, a serious physical diagnosis, and for all attending physicians, this book will move you deeply. It offers a wealth of insight into ways of approaching each step along the way, told through the mind and heart of a physician, now also a patient who is sharing what she is going through as it takes place. From breaking the news to spouse and children, to dealing with fears and mental projections, to listening to one's own needs and inner wisdom, this book makes the entire enterprise one of exploration and learning, as one deals with all the challenges that present themselves. This book is not about hiding from what's happening, but about allowing the experience of each step to teach you what you need to know as you go. It is the perfect example of the way in which life supports you when you are open and receptive, no matter the situation."

—Sarah Susanka, best-selling author of *The Not So Big House and The Not So Big Life* series

"After a breast cancer diagnosis lands her on the other side of the stethoscope, author Heather Thompson Buum writes with delightful candor about what happens when the doctor becomes the patient. Mirth is God's Medicine is an insightful, inspiring read for those of us looking for joy on some of life's most difficult journeys."

—Roxane Battle, former Kare 11 News Anchor and Author, *Pockets of Joy*

May this be the last time!

Mirth is God's Medicine

HEATHER THOMPSON BUUM, M.D.

Thank you for the support!
Heather

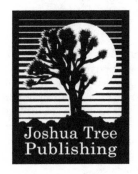

Joshua Tree
Publishing

• Chicago •

Mirth is God's Medicine
HEATHER THOMPSON BUUM, M.D.

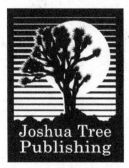

Published by
Joshua Tree Publishing
• Chicago •
JoshuaTreePublishing.com

13-Digit ISBN: 978-1-941049-52-5
Copyright © 2019. Heather Thompson Buum, MD All Rights Reserved.

Front Cover Image Credit: © cienpiesnf

Cover Background Image Credit: © THesIMPLIFY

Bible verses are from unless noted: New International Version (NIV)
Holy Bible, New International Version®, NIV® Copyright ©1973, 1978, 1984, 2011 by Biblica, Inc.® Used by permission. All rights reserved worldwide.

New American Standard Bible (NASB)
Copyright © 1960, 1962, 1963, 1968, 1971, 1972, 1973, 1975, 1977, 1995 by The Lockman Foundation

Printed in the United States of America

Mirth is God's medicine. Everybody ought to bathe in it. Grim care, moroseness, anxiety—all the rust of life—ought to be scoured off with the oil of mirth.

—Henry Ward Beecher

TABLE OF CONTENTS

Chapter 1

PROLOGUE

All bodies are transparent to this agent . . .
For the sake of brevity, I shall call them X-rays.
—Wilhelm Rontgen

I am lying on a gurney, a soft pink exam gown draped around my shoulders and tucked loosely into the top of my pants, perhaps to mimic some sense of modesty, I suppose. I've just had my first mammogram, followed by an ultrasound. The technicians for each test were both very nice, offering a friendly small talk. One of them asked if I had been to any baby showers lately—she's trying to plan one for her niece and needed to come up with games to play. I could not help but wonder at that time, Can they see the look on my face? Sense my fear? Are they trying anything to distract me? *Maybe there is no baby shower.*

I've been waiting now probably for twenty minutes but what seems like an eternity. The room is dark so that everyone can see the images on the screen. There is the sound of rushing air, a cooling fan for the equipment offering a soothing white noise. In the dim light, I can barely make out the framed prints on the wall; they appear to be garden scenes, impressionistic.

A soft knock, then a bright light pierces the dark. "I'm Dr. Rebecca Marsh," says the radiologist as she strides in, followed by another technician. Dr. Marsh is wearing blue scrubs and has chin-length, bobbed dark hair and funky square glasses. Turquoise, as I recall. She has a kind face, a soft smile.

I sit up on the gurney. "I'm an internal medicine doc," I tell her. "You can talk to me in technical terms, if need be." I want her to know she has permission to speak freely, to use the very shop talk we're all told to strictly avoid when speaking with patients.

I had never requested this in the past. When I was pregnant, I sought care at a health system outside from the one I worked in. I never told anyone I was a doctor, perhaps out of a need for privacy. But mostly, I didn't want anyone treating me any differently—I especially did not want them assuming I knew *anything* about pregnancy and delivery. As an internist, I gladly pushed ob-gyn and peds out of my brain to make room for diabetes, heart failure, and so on. Later, I found out that "physician" was all over my chart; somehow it had gotten through to them anyway. This time, I didn't care; I just wanted more information.

After my full disclosure, Dr. Marsh says, "Oh! Where do you practice?" I tell her at the University of Minnesota. "Really!" she says. "I'm a cancer survivor. The U saved my life! I absolutely love my doctors there. Dr. Rob Madoff, Dr. Anne Blaes—they are the best."

Wow. First, funny she should mention Anne Blaes. I had already thought of her when I pondered the lump I found days earlier. She's an outstanding oncologist, truly A team. But she's also a colleague of mine. We trained at the same residency program, just a few years apart—later, the two of us would collaborate on curriculum for the second year of medical school. It seems as though it might be strange now asking her to be my doctor.

Second, I'm struck by Dr. Marsh's immediate offering of very personal information. The lawyers call it PHI—protected health information. I'm impressed by her openness, her honesty. This was different from the "shop talk" I wanted when I let her know that I, too, was a doctor. I am immediately grateful, appreciative of her approach. *She understands what I am going through.*

Dr. Marsh interrupts my thoughts: "I'm afraid this looks like a cancer to me. I can biopsy it right here, right now, today, if you have time." I appreciate her forward approach and the blunt honesty—just what I'd asked for. I didn't want to hear: "Well, might be something, might not. Let's biopsy next week and wait for results." Radiologists who do this day in and day out must be able to tell right away when something looks suspicious. I would rather not skirt the issue.

So I say, yes, I have time and that I've cleared my schedule all afternoon. I am honestly not surprised. I knew immediately when I detected the lump at home that something wasn't right. I will say that leading up to the tests, I had a phrase running through my head: "Eighty percent of breast biopsies are benign." That is true and sounds like good enough odds for Vegas, right? But I admit, I had a feeling I was going to be in the 20 percent.

Dr. Marsh and the technician set immediately to work, bringing in trays in order to prep, drape, inject anesthesia, and sample. All the while, she is telling me the story of her cancer journey. It's not just colon cancer; it's metastatic colon cancer, diagnosed on a first screening colonoscopy at age fifty. It must have been a shock. She's had multiple surgeries, including mets removed from her liver, and goes in every week for chemotherapy. Dr. Marsh points out—as many patients have to me—that our new building feels so much different than the old building. I'm thinking, *Weekly chemo? Yet here she is, doing my biopsy—she is able to work.*

We exchange other stories: She also completed residency training at the U and talks about how crazy the schedule was for interventional radiology. I tell her that it still is, that nothing has changed, and that the pager goes off *constantly.* We laugh about the good old days when residency was fairly brutal, truly a rite of passage—this was prior to the residency duty-hour restrictions that occurred years later.

I tell Dr. Marsh I have never had a screening mammogram because there is "no data" to suggest a benefit for women under the age of fifty. "Don't get me started!" she says, her tone changing sharply. "I see just as many cancers in women in their forties. The guidelines are crap."

Which, in an odd way, is exactly how I found this lump. I had decided to forgo mammograms until later, but after I was done having kids and breastfeeding, I started to perform regular self-exams. I thought, *Well, gee-whiz, I'm a physician. I've been trained to do this. I should at least be checking myself at home.* Now keep in mind that the guidelines would also tell you there is "no evidence" for women to do self-exams. Go figure. I share this story with Dr. Marsh now, and we both have a laugh. I even tell her that I had just read through the *Annals of Internal Medicine,* February 2016. The entire issue was devoted to "solving the breast cancer screening controversies." After reviewing it cover to cover, I tossed it aside, frustrated, feeling no further along than before. Clear as mud. And now here I am, wading through it.

Dr. Marsh's technical expertise is very good—she's numbed the entire area, and I feel absolutely nothing even as this cap gun noise indicates the core biopsy is being taken. She asks me about my kids, their ages, and their hobbies and gives me advice about breaking the news to them. "I decided right away to involve their teachers at school," she says, "and that was a really great move." Her kids were older, though, teenagers—and I am worried about Lydia, who is nine, and Sam, twelve. I'm concerned that right away they will think I am dying. Other fears are rushing in as well: What does this mean for Lydia? I'm forty-four, not that young but not that old—could this be genetic? How good—*really*—is my health insurance plan? I've barely needed it before. What about life insurance, disability coverage? Time off work? Thoughts are tumbling in faster than I can respond to them.

"Do you know Dr. Sally Berryman?" Dr. Marsh asks. I snap out of it. Why yes, of course, she's a colleague of mine. We see patients side by side in the Primary Care Clinic. She also teaches essentials of clinical medicine, and I am a small group facilitator in that course. "What a coincidence! She's my primary physician. I am actually seeing her tomorrow at 10:00 a.m. I could be running into you there!"

Later on, she's holding pressure over the area to reduce any bleeding complications. At my teaching hospital, typically this is the job for the medical student. In the community private practice arena, it's her task. During this time, she's using those last few moments to comment once more on how I must seek care at the university. "You are a full-time physician? With two kids? Just being there on-site for appointments will save you time and energy you could use elsewhere." On the possibility that it might be awkward to be recognized: "You would be surprised. As a patient, the U is a pretty big place. You can sort of disappear if you want to." And once again: "You really need to see Anne Blaes."

After this last step is done and I return to the locker room to get dressed and gather my things, Dr. Marsh calls me back to her reading room to show me the mammogram images. There, projected on a very large screen, in the center of her desk, in full panoramic view, she points out the area that corresponded to the mass. I step in closer. I peer at it for a while, tilt my head, squint, back away, look again, and think, *Really?* I can barely make out anything. I turn to her, eyebrows raised; she says, "Honestly, I am not sure I would have even questioned this area, at all, if you had not told me there was something there. But the ultrasound confirmed what you were feeling." There is a background of extreme density; everything looks white to me. It's like trying to find a snowball in a blizzard.

I thank her again and, after shaking her hand, make my way out toward the lobby, emerging from darkness into the bright sunshine now filling the window-lined space. I am truly in a daze. I had spent about an hour and a half total with the radiologist, and I was there by myself that day—I didn't want my anxious husband pacing around the waiting room and me worrying about getting back to him. It was honestly about the most pleasant ninety minutes I could ask for, considering the circumstances. Having these conversations with another female physician, a few steps ahead of me on a similar journey, gave me a perspective I could not *possibly* have imagined from time spent in a radiology suite. From her expert opinion to the sharing of anecdotes, to the sage advice and personal recommendations, I was getting complimentary life coaching along with my diagnostic procedure. A harbinger of things to come, perhaps—a taste of what it might be like, going forward, as a doctor about to become patient. I sat in my car in the parking lot for a long time afterward, contemplating the enormity of it.

The next day, I was back in the clinic, with a full schedule of my own patients. My chest was sore and had a bit of bruising; I winced if the bell of my stethoscope hit just the wrong area. Earlier that morning, I rummaged around in my old antique secretary desk at home and wrote a thank-you card for Dr. Marsh: "Thank you for your kind and compassionate care of me yesterday, in addition to your technical expertise. And thank you so much for sharing your story with me; it gave me hope and courage."

In the clinic's computer workspace known as the collaboration zone, I walked over and sat down next to Dr. Sally Berryman. Slipping her the card—addressed to Dr. Rebecca Marsh on the front of the envelope—I said cheerfully, "Please give this to your 10:20 patient." Sally looked down. "Oh! It's Becky. I haven't seen her in while!" Then she looks up at me, a puzzled expression on her face. "I'll explain later." And off I went to see my next patient.

* * *

As time went on, I would reflect back on this interaction with Dr. Marsh and realize how it was the starting point, the moment I began to fundamentally shift my perspective as a doctor. Dr. Marsh's openness and my ensuing experiences as a patient would give me the courage to try a new approach in my practice—that there can be intrinsic value in transparency, in sharing one's story with others. Even private, personal, sometimes painful stories. Making connections and creating a bond can be the ultimate expression of empathy—it's important for patients to know that physicians experience the same things they do, including the fear, turmoil, and strife that is a part of becoming a patient in our complicated system. Over time, I kept finding remarkable ways in which being in one role benefitted the other.

As I began to write—telling stories not just about me, my health, my medical situation but also about how it changed me as a person, a friend, a spouse, a parent, a teacher, a doctor—I began to think, *Perhaps others might benefit from reading this book.* Just as I did from hearing Dr. Marsh's story. Writing also became a new outlet for me; it was just as they say, "Cheaper than therapy," and a coping mechanism for dealing with a new diagnosis in addition to what had sustained me previously—music, faith, fitness, and a sense of humor. In fact, I found many instances of humor throughout this endeavor—who can endure the unforgettable experience of having a breast MRI without reflecting back on the ridiculousness of it all? And hopefully, laughing about it at some point. Because as the verse says in Proverbs: "A cheerful heart is good medicine." There is something very healing about the ability to laugh and find humor in these dark situations.

But mostly, I appreciated the incredible opportunity to connect with my patients on a much deeper level. Perhaps the gift of writing will increase the impact—adding to, expanding upon, and deepening those connections even more. Even prior to this, the goal of any type of writing endeavor in my career thus far has been to have someone else read and benefit from it, such as publishing results from a mentoring program or an educational innovation. Hopefully, someone else would learn from it, gain insight, or take something away they could use back at their home institution. And that is certainly true of this book as well. While I sincerely hope no one would have to endure a cancer diagnosis in order to become a better doctor, a better teacher, and so on, the truth of the matter is, we will all be patients someday. Taking time to pause and reflect and explore the borders between the two is a meaningful and worthwhile endeavor. And taking time to read about it might make us all better in these roles as well.

Chapter 2

THE ROLLER COASTER

Your life is like a roller coaster, baby, that I don't want to ride.
—Ohio Players, "Love Rollercoaster"
(with a few edits by me)

I n the early weeks after my diagnosis, I had a lot of thoughts, phrases, even songs racing through my mind. Clichés, for the most part. "What doesn't kill you makes you stronger"—that sort of thing. But for some reason, it was that '70s Ohio Players tune "Love Rollercoaster" covered in the 1990s by the Red Hot Chili Peppers that kept playing in my mind. I know it's a trite analogy, but it stuck—the ups and downs, twists and turns. Only this ride was a little too crazy for me, so I altered the lyrics a bit to suit my situation.

The mid-1990s is probably the last time I actually tuned into pop music consistently enough to know that the Red Hot Chili Peppers remade that song. I had graduated from college in 1993, took one year off to do research, then started medical school in the fall of 1994. After that, it is a bit of a blur, to be honest. Not that I didn't enjoy it—I can honestly say I loved medical school. I felt as though I could finally learn what I was supposed to be learning as opposed to, say, differential equations in calculus. But it really does consume your entire life. The first two years, studying every possible moment of the day, memorizing innervation, origin, insertion of each muscle in the human body, along with biochemistry, genetics, later pharmacology, pathology—it's just like they say, *taking a drink from a fire hose*. Then in the third and fourth years, you are on clinical rotations, and your time is not your own. Show up at 5:30 a.m. for rounds? Sure! Lecture at 8:00 a.m. on a Saturday? Great!

So it was funny that my mind went back to that era in my life; in some ways, it was crazy, even more hectic, but in other ways much more simple—because your life and your schedule is essentially dictated for you. And the other funny thing is, even at my age, I still love roller coasters. My family of four—including my petite but brave girl who barely clears the height restrictions—has ridden every coaster at Valleyfair, our favorite being Wild Thing. We've experienced the Rip Ride Rocket at Universal, the Expedition Everest at Disney, the Raging Bull at Six Flags—the list goes on. Maybe that's why this analogy fits so well for me.

Hill number 1:

I find out I have not one but *two* foci of cancer in my right breast, and immediately, my mind jumps to the fact that I will probably need a mastectomy, not a lumpectomy, and then lightning fast from there, what if I need a bilateral mastectomy due to genetics? Hey! I could get a free boob job! As a gal who has been an A cup all my life, I could go B or even C—how great is that?

Drop number 1:

Oh, but wait: multiple steps, many procedures. Tissue expanders. Chest wall pain. Pectoralis muscle weakness. One of my patients developed an infection at the tissue expander site and had to go in for a washout, IV antibiotics, and then start the entire process all over again. Potential complications, down, down, down. I know right then and there, in a span of about thirty seconds, that reconstruction was not for me. No surgery if it's not medically necessary. After all, I start to reason, an A cup is not much different than a perfectly flat chest. I'll get used to it; I'll wear padded bras the rest of my life. And even after much more careful consideration and many discussions, eventually I stick by that decision.

Hill number 2:

I am going to meet with a genetic counselor to go over my family history and decide on genetic testing. I tell her ahead of time that this is going to be a very short, boring meeting—I only know half my family history. I do not know my biological father, and there is really no cancer on my mother's side. I've already made up my mind to go ahead and order the testing, but the actual appointment seems like a waste of time.

Drop number 2:

I talk on the phone with Mom, who reminds me that she has spoken with a friend of my biological father at one time who said that, apparently, he was diagnosed with prostate cancer at least ten years ago, placing him in his early fifties at the time of diagnosis. Then it dawns on me: the BRCA mutation is associated with prostate cancer, as well as breast and ovarian. It's the Sherlock Holmes aspect of medicine that we all love—trying to put together the clues and figure out why something is happening. *Aha! BRCA!* Elementary, my dear Watson (and Crick!).

Oh, but wait. Ovarian as well as breast—I might need a gyn-onc surgeon as well, or at least an ultrasound and CA-125 blood test every six months. Then I flash to my children, Lydia and Sam. Sam, who at twelve is already taller than me and experiencing the surges of testosterone—the oily hair, the mild acne, the changing voice, the mood swings. And prostate cancer is a testosterone-dependent tumor. I think of that hormone just starting to course through his veins and consider the long-term implications, a possible need for screening, biopsies, surgeries, or more. And Lydia—it's not just the prophylactic mastectomy. Angelina Jolie has made that option not only understandable but downright noble and/or some sort of a feminist statement—it's about fertility implications. Surgical removal of both ovaries by age thirty-five? I had not even had my second child at that point. I want to be a grandma someday! All these thoughts, again in a span of about thirty seconds, and knowing full well I won't even hear the results of this genetic testing for *weeks*. This was a tough drop, leaving me breathless at the bottom, just like Wild Thing.

Hill number 3:

My blood pressure. Another bit of a ride, with ups and down that mirrored my current state of anxiety; and after all, every coaster has its small side hills. I was diagnosed with high blood pressure about six months before I learned I had cancer. It had been "borderline" for a while, but with a strong family history, I knew I'd be on meds someday. I was started on an ace inhibitor, then developed the most annoying cough, and was switched to an angiotensin receptor blocker. Needless to say, on a tiny dose of this medication, it was well controlled—until I started going in for multiple appointments to work up the breast mass. At my first office visit after I had found the lump, it was sky-high, 160 over 100 or something crazy like that. At the surgeon's office, the first reading was almost as bad; the second came down to 140s over 90s. Still, my primary doctor sees it and mentions it and suggests I go up on my medication. First, increase the ARB dose, then add a diuretic.

Drop number 3:

A week or two after these changes, it's a Saturday. I get up, have some breakfast, then make a quick trip to the grocery store. I'm unloading items in the kitchen, bending over to place something on a lower shelf, stand up, and *whoa* . . . the entire room goes dim, almost black. Feeling woozy, I immediately go to the table and sit down, and after taking a few sips of water, I start feeling better. I get my home blood pressure cuff and check: 94/64. What? Take it again: 100/68. After I recover, I walk into the bathroom and look at my new medication in its prescription bottle. I had just filled this combination tablet, darn it, ninety of them; I didn't want to get a new or different Rx. I pop out one of the little round peach tablets. Aha, they are scored; I can split the dose in half. I decide to start doing that without telling anyone as I really don't want to make another call to the doctor, relay a message, and play phone tag. And hey, now the prescription will last me twice as long! Bonus! As you can see, physicians are not all that different from patients. We don't always follow instructions to the letter. And it just goes to show you how very different blood pressure readings are at home compared to the medical office.

Hill number 4:

The emotions. Of course, this one is obvious. I just found that I had such strange, almost idiosyncratic reactions at times. During the week, taking care of patients, teaching students and residents, I did great. I felt this new, incredibly strong connection with the health-care system, including my patients. And it was really gratifying. I could look a patient in the eye who had a newly diagnosed cancer and honestly say I knew how they felt. This connection was truly a soaring high for me. And for some odd reason, I also looked forward to having additional tests. You need to draw labs? Another MRI? *When can I be there?* You think genetic testing should be done? Let's check not just BRCA but that panel of seventeen mutations screening for everything under the sun. I can only imagine that this is the physician in me needing more information, wanting to move forward, come up with the treatment plan. Although in my own practice, I actually tend to *avoid* ordering too many tests, so this seemed very unlike me. Sometimes, I felt strangely energized, even elated—this cancer is not taking me down!

Drop number 4:

The lows usually came in the evenings or on the weekends, when I had more time to think things through. I found myself waking up at 2:00 or 3:00 a.m. and staring at the ceiling. At that point, I could take a half tablet of Benadryl and usually fall back asleep. It was much worse if I woke up at 4:00 a.m. because that was really too late to take anything. After a certain hour, it was more staring at the ceiling, more thinking, more prayer time, followed by lots of coffee to get me through. Once on a low day, I thought, *If every day is a gift from God, I certainly don't want to spend every day feeling like this. When am I going to get any joy back?* I would look at family photos taken just weeks ago on a spring break vacation and marvel at the carefree expression on my face.

But for the most part, I didn't feel depressed, just at times extremely anxious, stressed, agitated, irritable, and really distracted. I recall one time working in my office on my computer, and when somebody knocked on my door, I jumped out of my skin, actually letting out a small shout. I opened the door, and it was my course manager, Jeff, standing there with wide eyes. I just mumbled, "Sorry, I have a lot going on right now," or something lame like that. I also recall dropping my kids off at school one morning and then driving right back to my house—when I was supposed to drive into work. I began to wonder if I should be seeing patients in my distracted state of mind.

On the other hand, this was basically how I felt for most of 1998 to 2001, when I was a resident on call every fourth night. On the "post call" day, up most of the night and sleep-deprived, I was still expected to carry out all the usual job duties the next day and sometimes into the evening. My record: staying until 10:00 p.m. the next evening after a horrific night in the Regions ICU—that's forty hours straight without sleeping. Back then, I did not consider this unusual; I felt somehow that my reflexes took over, and what I had learned in medicine was so ingrained that I could function on autopilot.

Come to think of it, that wasn't just residency—Sam and Lydia were not great sleepers in their first years of life, and after being up at least two to three times a night with them (and *every* night, not every fourth night) over several months, I began to feel the same way. We now have residency duty-hour restrictions; too bad the same doesn't apply for motherhood.

And now here I was again, years later, relying on autopilot but for an entirely different reason. And while sleep deprivation feels a whole heck of a lot worse at age forty-four, I now had many more years of clinical experience to rely upon. At times, I feel like I can just look at a patient and tell how sick they are. Somehow, despite lack of sleep or other distractions, it still works. It sounds crazy, I know, but it's how we as physicians function. At one point, I reflect on the irony—that this sort of training is helping me continue on, to keep working as a doctor while experiencing the stress of becoming a patient.

So after that "Love Rollercoaster" song gets stuck in my mind, I decided to embrace it. I thought I might even have it on an old compilation CD, *Pure Disco*. Yes, I am *really* dating myself here; I still have all my music collection on CDs. So I pop it in on the way to work, find the song on track 11, and smile as the familiar tune fills the car.

And in a similar fashion, I started to embrace the roller-coaster ride as it pertains to the cancer diagnosis. There are constant ups and downs, twists and turns. You are never quite sure where the ride is going; all you know is that you are strapped in—and you are hoping the car doesn't go off the rails. Letting out a big scream once in a while helps too. Those universal safety instructions also come to mind: "Keep your hands and feet inside the car at all times. Please remain seated until the ride comes to a complete stop."

Then I pause and think, *Complete stop. To where exactly is this ride taking me?*

Chapter 3

THE SEARCH FOR A SURGEON

The reputation of a surgeon, in the final analysis, must
rest upon originality, teaching by word of mouth,
teaching by printed word, and operative skill.
—William J. Mayo

After the biopsy but before the results were back, I found myself contemplating the fact that I would need surgery for the first time in my life. *Ever.* I started to wonder— how do people go about choosing a surgeon? Even someone like me, armed with a fair amount of baseline medical knowledge?

Most women likely ask their primary care doctor for a recommendation. I am sure many also search Google or perhaps look at those dubious doctor rating websites or even Angie's List. Here in Minnesota, we have two magazines—*Mpls St Paul* and *Minnesota Monthly*—that every year list the Twin Cities' Top Doctors as selected by their peers. It has, of course, come under fire for being a popularity contest, a ranking that is not evidence-based or linked to outcomes. However, every year I look at that list myself and think, *Yeah, they're pretty spot-on.* I recognize many names that I would feel very confident referring a family member to. Or in this case, myself.

I spent pretty much an entire weekend searching. I began to realize that even as a general internist—I already knew quite a bit about hormonal therapy (tamoxifen), and I've been to grand rounds, discussing targeted chemotherapy (Herceptin)—the weak spot in my own knowledge was the surgical management of this disease. *It's the surgeon whose expertise I really need to rely upon, so I'd better choose wisely.* The name of Dr. Todd Tuttle had come immediately to mind the moment the radiologist said it looked suspicious. But then I thought, *Well, that's because he is at the U, and his name is all over the EMR.* I've referred patients to him myself; I've done many of his preops, hopefully to his satisfaction—although I secretly suspect no surgeon ever reads them.

And so I began my search in earnest—and not with Google but with PubMed. A search by author returned over one hundred articles by Todd M. Tuttle. Impressive! Many of them were regarding breast cancer; several were for melanoma, appendiceal cancer, and more. I was intrigued by some of the titles: "Bilateral Mastectomy: Doubling Down on Complications?" or "Contralateral Prophylactic Mastectomy: Are We Overtreating Patients?" *Good,* I thought, *he's not afraid to take on some of the controversial issues.* In fact, the more I read, the more confident I grew that he might be a good fit. After I defaulted back to Google, I saw how well-known and respected Dr. Todd Tuttle truly was. There were many public accolades to be found, interviews on CNN, videos on YouTube, awards, endowed chairs for research. And yes, of course, he made that Top Docs' list. Pretty much every year.

I did go on to research many more surgeons, literally all across the Twin Cities—the Jane Brattain Breast Center at Park Nicollet, Hennepin County Medical Center, the Piper Breast Center at Abbott, North Memorial. But then, I began to think about my life—working full-time, with two children, activities, hobbies. Why drive halfway across town for appointments when I could walk down the hall in the same building and consult with expertise of this level? The advice from my radiologist, Dr. Marsh, echoed back. Yet it did still give me pause, to think of becoming a patient in my own system. Would it feel awkward divulging all my personal history, family history, medical history, and God knows what else going forward? But of course, even from the MD perspective, the U is a very big place. There are over 750 doctors in the practice of University of Minnesota Physicians. There are "colleagues" of mine I probably would not recognize if I saw them at a shopping mall or a sporting event.

Also, I am struck by how much reading through an extensive list of publications can give any patient a keen sense of the mind-set of the authoring physician. I'm very much in favor of evidence-based medicine, the idea of exercising restraint—not "doing" something just because we can or think we should or the patient is demanding it—that's right in line with my personal philosophy, my practice style. Many of Dr. Tuttle's papers reflected that same approach. I couldn't really get that feel regarding any other surgeon I researched, and I began to think, how do people select a doctor *without* this kind of information? How would one choose a surgeon, a specialist, a primary care physician? You might schedule the appointment, meet them, realize it's not a good fit, and then have to start all over, wasting time, energy, even money. I started to think, huh, maybe our dean is onto something. He's been pushing us harder to publish our scholarly work, even educational endeavors. I'm recognizing it might be much more than just good PR for the university.

Early the following week, I get a call at 8:00 a.m. that the biopsy is positive for cancer. I spend a few minutes hyperventilating—literally—and then start to think, *I've got to calm down. I've got work to do.* After the initial shock wears off a bit, an hour later I call my husband with the news, then e-mail him a link to Dr. Tuttle's bio on the M Health website. He replies back: "I like him. Looks like he's done this before." Now, I know Paul is an architect, but still, the carte blanche endorsement gives me a boost of confidence. He has also been saying from the very beginning that I should go to the U. This is how the locals view things: for the best medical care, it's either the U or Mayo. And even though, of course, I'm biased, I think it's correct.

Around noon, I dial the call center in an attempt to schedule an appointment. I get placed on hold for an inordinate amount of time and hang up. I must admit, I am not the most patient person to begin with, and at a time like this, I am certainly not in the best state of mind for the entire phone-tree/on-hold-music experience. I'm pacing around my living room, contemplating calling back or trying a more direct number to the clinic. But instead, I give up, put the phone back on the cradle, go to my home computer, and log into the EMR. I send what is called a staff message to Dr. Tuttle.

"Hello, I am an internist in Primary Care. I have recently been diagnosed with breast cancer. I am wondering if you would take me on as a patient. I tried to go through the call center with not much luck. If you would like me to speak with your nurse or someone else, please let me know."

I drive into work much later than I normally would, eventually heading over to the clinic when I get a call on my cell from Dr. Tuttle's nurse, Susan. He added me on at 7:30 a.m. the very next day. I breathe a huge sigh of relief; just knowing I have that appointment is such a strong encouragement. I can hardly believe it. It's my first of many experiences, thinking, wow, this is what we put our patients through—dialing impersonal call centers, going through phone trees, filling out intake forms, leaving messages that are not returned for days when all we really want to hear is that one simple phrase, "Yes, the doctor will see you."

If there is *any* reason God is allowing this to happen in my life, this realization very well may be one of them.

Chapter 4

BREAKING BAD (PART I)

Hide what you have to hide, tell what you have to tell.
—Depeche Mode, "The Policy of Truth"

All physicians receive training on how to deliver bad news to a patient. We were taught a specific five-step process, even practicing via role play, video, using actors as fake patients, and so on. Still, I don't think I ever appreciated how difficult it truly was until I tried to apply it to my own family.

Following my diagnosis, I had a hard time deciding how exactly to break the news to Paul because I wasn't really sure how he would take it. He tends to be a rather anxious person. And I don't just mean a worrier personality type; yes, there's that, but there have also been flare-ups, two episodes in our marriage where the anxiety became more of an issue, more disabling. And this was when everything was going great! We were healthy. Our kids were doing well in school. We both enjoyed our work. Financially, we were stable. The list goes on. I guess that is why it is called *generalized anxiety disorder*—there is no specific reason for the anxiety. It just generally *is*.

So I find myself thinking and worrying that when I tell Paul I have breast cancer, he could potentially go into another tailspin. At times, I sense the anxiety is simply at a low simmer, just below the surface. Another boil-over—well, I'm not sure I can handle that right now. During the last episode, I tried to be the helpful spouse and figure out ways to support him, help him through it; but now, at this point in time, I feel I have just enough to get *me* through the day.

In the early days, right after the abnormal mammogram, oh, how I wanted so much to just fall apart and have someone else take care of me. I was so tired of holding everything up on my own. I had felt this way another time before when battling colic with my two-month-old son Sam every night and, I believe, in retrospect, some untreated postpartum depression. I became very sleep-deprived and so stressed by him crying every single night for hours on end. I recall that it was early November 2004, because we stayed up way too late watching the election results even long after Sam was *finally* asleep. Early November in Minnesota is also extremely edgy—daylight is dying, cold settling in, wind blowing around the few straggling leaves left on the ground, the excitement of the holidays not quite here yet, no sparkling white snow, just dead brown and dreary. I thought I was going to lose my mind.

At one point, I had this highly irrational thought: Why can't I get appendicitis or a low-grade diverticulitis or a mild case of pneumonia, something not *that* serious but where I could get admitted to the hospital for a few days, just have the nurses take care of me, and I can hand off this baby and I might actually get some sleep? Come to think of it, I might not even need to *have* any of these things; I could simply get admitted for observation. I thought this through to the highest level: I will present to the ER, knowing exactly what to say. I can probably even fake some right lower quadrant pain with peritoneal signs. Is this crazy or what? But understandable, in retrospect. Luckily, it never came to that. The colic abruptly ceased at around four months. It left with no explanation other than my pediatrician's suggestion it might have been acid reflux.

This time around, I realize fairly quickly I can't fall apart no matter how much I want to. I have my family—and my own patients—who still need me. Thank God it's April and not November; the weather is definitely in my favor. And even the anxiety of a cancer diagnosis is not quite as mind-altering as my postpartum state, believe it or not.

As far as sharing the news with Paul, I brainstorm exactly how to do this, and I decide I'm going to try it on a need-to-know basis, offering information just one piece at a time and only what we *know*, not what is unknown. I will try not to mention results that are "pending" and instead wait so we can have an actual result to discuss, not just theoretical possibilities. Why spend the extra days waiting, worrying? I'll do enough of that for the two of us, thank you.

This approach, while initially sounds great, totally backfires. To start, I didn't even tell Paul until the morning of the appointment that I am having a mammogram—and possibly a biopsy—even though this all started *days* ago, including an office visit with my primary MD, who confirmed the lump with a furrowed brow, and I knew immediately that she was concerned as well. But the day of the radiology appointment, Paul's actually nonchalant. "Well, if you found a lump, yes, you should go get it checked out." I think, wow, he has no idea that I know this is going to be abnormal. I must be hiding it pretty well! Strong work! I then tell Paul, "Most breast biopsies turn out benign." I am trying not to add to his anxiety even though I was totally convinced otherwise myself. He agrees with me and seems reassured, and now, for a split second, I am almost . . . offended that he is *not* more concerned. But better that than the opposite, I guess. Five days later, after I got the call that the biopsy was positive, I *did* tell him that news almost immediately but didn't expand further other than to say I will need surgery and maybe chemotherapy or radiation. The next steps are TBD.

As time went on, though, I had a hard time keeping track of which studies I have told him about versus those I haven't. Do I bother telling him about genetic testing that takes weeks to return or just wait until the actual result is available? It turns out to be too long of a wait. I simply can't hold it in, and start complaining about how a completely erroneous test was ordered initially, a CA-27.29, some tumor marker, which led to even further delays for the actual needed result. The same thing occurs later on with conflicting imaging studies. *Why are you having yet another MRI?* Oh, crap, I wasn't going to mention that; now the cat is out of the bag. While I am trying to spare him the fear and anxiety that accompanies the unknown, now he's just getting frustrated, thinking I'm not being truthful or I'm withholding information from him. I can't blame him; essentially, I am.

I would do this again one last time while waiting on what is called the oncotype assay, a test run on the tumor itself that helps predict the risk of recurrence. I'm in a holding pattern, pining away, waiting with bated breath, knowing this basically determines whether or not I will need chemo—but I don't even mention it to Paul until after the fact, after its return, which took quite some time.

And exactly why I'm doing all this, I'm not so sure. Overall, he is coping much better than I expected. He didn't seem nearly as stressed as I thought he would be—no major tailspin—just at times, a general avoidance of the topic. Not that he didn't want to be helpful, but being a physician myself, it was essentially "Honey, you're the doctor, do whatever you think is best." *But I'm not the doctor, I am the patient!* Having complete deference to my opinion on the treatment plan, on some level it's great—but on another level, *what? You don't care that my right breast will be gone forever with nothing in its place?*

I keep these thoughts to myself. I'm picking up on his cues that perhaps his coping mechanism is somewhat akin to the ostrich approach. *Stick your head in the sand and wait until this whole thing blows over.* Other than the day of surgery itself—I needed a driver, after all!—he doesn't attend any appointments. I mention the dates and times but don't push the issue; I didn't insist that he come, but I didn't tell him not to, either. Once, prior to my first oncology visit, I started to talk about it, listing the questions I had. He interrupts me and says something to the effect of "Save it for the appointment." I just clam up immediately and slowly nod.

But then I wonder, starting to get concerned, Who does *he* have to talk with, to vent about this? Me, I've got all these support networks, circles of female friends, from church to my kid's school to the choir I've been a part of for twenty years. I suggest multiple times that he talk to Troy, his friend from architecture school and best man in our wedding. His wife, Michelle, was diagnosed with breast cancer two years ago. To this day, I'm not sure if he ever did. The two of us seem to be handling it in completely opposite ways, neither being better or worse. Just different. Part of me wonders if this is somehow the stereotypical male-versus-female response.

It was around this time that I started to write about my experiences to harness the therapeutic effects of writing. I've done this before. As an associate program director for the internal medicine residency at the University of Minnesota, I met with a subset of residents every six months. I conducted a semi-annual review, where I would not only evaluate their performance but also assess for fatigue, stress, burnout—that sort of thing. I worked with one resident more extensively, a young man struggling in several areas, including communication skills. Not knowing exactly how to make the situation better, I think I was able to finally engage him by having him write, mostly composing essays, reflective pieces.

I recall a particularly poignant short story he gave to me, an experience about losing a young patient with lupus and a complex medical history to overwhelming sepsis after encountering a delay in antibiotics. I also learned that he was out on a five-mile run near the university when the I-35W bridge collapsed, and he arrived on the scene, trying to help as a physician. This ongoing writing went on for the entire duration of his residency, but I enjoyed taking this on, a project of sorts. After following through on assignments, meeting frequently, talking things over, the situation really did improve over time, a success story. I do believe that the writing exercises had a positive impact, allowing him to process some of the incredibly tough stuff that is part of medical training.

So this is how writing is for me as well; it's helping me process everything. It will save me from needing to unload onto Paul, sparing him additional anxiety. And at the end of the day, cancer is, more so than any other condition, an intensely personal diagnosis. You can talk with people, even medical professionals, ask for advice, read all the statistics you want, or look up information all day long—I think I could have broken the internet early on with my sheer number of Google and PubMed searches. But it's more about processing, assimilating, internalizing, synthesizing. Personalizing that information, figuring out how it applies to *you*, how it changes *your* outlook on life, and how it affects *your* future. That is something you can really only do for yourself, not relying on anyone else to do it for you; and the entire process, well, it simply takes time.

A lot of time, actually.

In fact, I began to think that writing was my personal way of breaking bad news *to myself.* Getting my thoughts, fears, emotions, and observations out of my brain and onto paper was extremely therapeutic. Seeing words on a page also made it feel more concrete, as if yes, this is actually happening—because at times it felt surreal. Thankfully, it was also moving me in the direction where I could get past the anxiety and pause, reflect, learn from—and therefore be changed by—my experiences as a patient.

The last two steps of breaking bad news are "Respond to their feelings" and "Plan the follow through." Later, coming back to my writing, rereading, expanding the text, developing themes, editing if you will—in a sense it was accomplishing the very same goal. It helped me respond to my own feelings and develop my plan, my own strategy going forward.

Interesting. Maybe writing should be included in that five-step approach.

Chapter 5

Breaking Bad (Part II)

1. Fire a warning shot.
2. Find out what they know.
3. Share information.
4. Respond to their feelings.
5. Plan the follow through.

In medical school, I learned the above five-step model on how to deliver bad news to a patient. I still fall back on this method time and again in my primary care clinic; I've even used it when giving really tough feedback to a learner who is struggling in some aspect of their performance. But I honestly never thought I would be applying these steps to my own children—breaking the news that Mom has breast cancer.

At this point, it's been one week since the biopsy returned positive for cancer. I've told my husband the news. I've had my appointments with surgery and oncology. I am starting to get a better sense of the plan. It seems like now is the time to let our children in on the situation, but naturally, I am feeling nervous.

I sought advice from several friends who were physicians and also parents themselves; I did get some helpful suggestions. "Tell them just enough information and not too much; let them ask the questions." My radiologist who was diagnosed with metastatic colon cancer at age fifty—yes, on first screening colonoscopy—she told me to involve their teachers at school and to be blunt, honest, and direct. Her kids were older, though, teenagers. What about Sam and Lydia, aged eight and eleven? After talking it over with

Paul, an architect, he thought I should lead the discussion and maybe appropriately so; we both reasoned I had the background medical knowledge and the training in this particular skill set that would hopefully come in handy.

The opportunity to have the talk arose on a Thursday evening, right after parent-teacher conferences. As part of Sam's fifth-grade conference, he was given an assignment to write about what he is learning, what he enjoys most, and goals for the next quarter. I had just seen this document; it was meant to prompt the discussion for those fifteen minutes of time with his teacher. On this, he had written "The Cell" as one of his most enjoyable learning topics. *Aha.* This might be a good way to open the conversation. I called them both into the kitchen; I am sure they thought this was going to be some sort of debrief about report cards or test scores.

I am standing at the counter, fixing dinner—shrimp diablo, a spicy tomato sauce with shrimp over pasta. It gets quite a bit of heat from a full two tablespoons of chili paste. My son likes the spice; my daughter typically douses it with parmesan to make it more palatable. "So parent-teacher conferences went well!" I say. I am trying to act casual as I am peeling the raw shrimp for use in the pasta. Their flimsy crustacean shells and odd-shaped legs fling down into the metal colander as I work while Sam and Lydia are sitting at the kitchen table. I turn to Sam and ask, "What do you know about the cell?"

"Well, you know, the cell is the building block of the human body. Every part of us is made up of cells." Indeed, I say, how fascinating, the nucleus, ribosomes, mitochondria. "What do you know about cancer?" I ask. (*Find out what they know.*) Sam says, "Cancer is when cells grow out of control and, like, take over your body and spread and stuff." Very good, I think. Our education dollars are going somewhere.

"Well, along those lines, I am afraid that your mom has something to tell you." (*Warning shot.*) "I found a lump in my breast. My doctors did a biopsy and discovered it is cancer."

I pause, swallow hard. I try not to mince words, but maybe this is too much. I will never forget the looks on their faces. Sam sits silent, and his pale blue eyes with their long sandy blond lashes simply widen—visibly widen—and he just freezes, staring back at me. Then Lydia, her beautiful hazel eyes and dark lashes just turn red and immediately fill with tears.

I go on to say, I know this sounds very frightening, but I am quite fortunate, I found this lump early. I tell them I'm seeking care at the university, to have the best physicians on board, the A team. I will have surgery to remove it, followed by medicine to control it. And I feel fine! This is the best possible scenario! It's a very treatable disease, I say. (*Share information.*)

At which point, Sam asks, "But is it curable?" Darn it, too smart for his own good.

I answer, "Yes, it is potentially curable."

"But could it come back?" Wow. Well, I say, that is a very good question. In theory, it could come back, but the medicine helps prevent that from happening. Lydia is still shedding tears and asking if my arms and legs feel weak from cancer. I am trying to reassure her; I tell her no, I am still running and I can still go on bike rides with her. Sam says, "Well, at least you are able to keep doing what you want to do." What is this, a future oncologist commenting on functional status? I cannot believe I am hearing these responses.

We exchange hugs, talk a bit more. I tell them it's perfectly normal to feel sad or scared and, of course, I do too, but I have complete trust in my team of doctors. (*Respond to their feelings.*) Eventually, we sit down to eat. I mention over dinner, if it helps, they can tell their friends at school, and I will speak with their parents or talk to their teachers if they would like them to know. (*Plan the follow through.*) Later, before bed, we all pray together about it.

But over the coming days, Sam pretty much clams up about the topic. He doesn't mention it, doesn't tell his friends, and doesn't need me to talk with his teacher, Mrs. Horn. Lydia, on the other hand, tells her two best friends; and they tell two friends and so on. She informs not only her current third-grade teacher but her beloved second-grade teacher as well. She's a very artsy, creative girl. She loves to draw; she and her classmates design a colorful "get well" card for me at school. Later, I find out Sam is keeping a journal and writes a few entries regarding the cancer diagnosis. This I'm glad to know; writing can be extremely therapeutic. It is interesting and a bit heartwarming to see how each of them processes the information—neither being better or worse, just different. Eerily similar to how Paul and I respond differently to the same situation.

In fact, after the initial panic, Lydia suddenly shifts gears and becomes almost my home visiting nurse. Every day, she wants to know how I am feeling, asks me if there is any pain, if I have eaten enough today, if I have gotten any exercise, when my other tests are coming back—I kid you not. Along a similar vein, she actually asks me, "Can I feel your lump?" I am really conflicted about that. What should I do? Am I going to warp an eight-year-old girl for the rest of her life? This is pretty scary stuff. I recall my early denial, when I kept feeling this lump for several days, hoping it would somehow miraculously disappear. Maybe it's just a fluid-filled cyst or something. I kept palpating to see if it was really there until I finally made the call to the clinic.

Eventually, I decide, well, why not? It might help to have some sort of tangible explanation of what is going on. She presses in where I had originally felt it; it's quite superficial, at "one o'clock" as they say, just above my bra line, fairly obvious. After the biopsy, there was a bit of swelling. Now it seems bigger than when I originally discovered it (or is that my imagination?). She does feel it right away and makes a perfect face: a cross between a frown and an expression of disgust, best described simply as "eeeww."

I couldn't agree more. It's yucky. It's gross. I can't wait to get rid of it.

Chapter 6

PREPARATION

Therefore do not worry about tomorrow, for
tomorrow will worry about itself. Each day has
enough trouble of its own.
—Matthew 6:34

I'm trying to keep my sanity and preserve both my mental and physical health for what I perceive is going to be a long journey ahead of me.

I realize, coming soon, after the operation—whatever surgical approach that may be—I am simply not going to be able to do as much for a while. No running for some time, no heavy lifting, certainly not swinging a golf club, and I have just finished watching the Masters on television, which heralds the beginning of the golf season. Here in Minnesota, we are having an unusually warm early spring, which is both a blessing and a curse. I look ahead, a bit frantically, trying to think of ways to book a tee time and get a babysitter so Paul and I can play a round of golf on the weekend. But despite the encouraging weather and seeing the amazing display of wisteria and azalea televised at Augusta, I discover once again what a head game golf truly is. I play nine holes with Paul one late afternoon, and given my high level of anxiety, it is an absolute disaster. My state of distraction is amazing; I am stepping up to a par 3, eighty yards out and pulling out my driver, even taking a practice swing before I realize this is the wrong club. My putting is all over the map. Midway through the round, I just stop keeping score, and I think of that Mark Twain quote, "Golf is a good walk, spoiled." Ironically, Paul is having the best round of his life. He finishes three over par. I think, wait, I thought *he* was the one with the anxiety issue!

Well, at least running does not require quite the same level of mental focus or mental stamina to continue to reap the benefits. In fact, it's almost the opposite; I can completely zone out and clear my mind of all the clutter. So I feel this pressure to run every morning up until the point I can no longer do it even though I know it's temporary. It's as if this clock is ticking up until the point of surgery, and although it's not exactly rational—I'm not losing a limb for God's sake!—I can't help but overdo it. I have been known to say, even before this diagnosis, that a three-mile run is my Xanax.

I also have little to no appetite. My stomach feels, most of the time, in knots. I will go until two thirty in the afternoon before I realize I haven't eaten anything. This is so unlike me; I enjoy cooking and going out to restaurants—I really *like* to eat. That, coupled with the increased exercise, and I have dropped six pounds in two weeks without even trying. Believe me, I do not recommend a new cancer diagnosis as a weight-loss strategy; on the other hand, I will admit, how much did I enjoy fitting into my skinny jeans again! Wow, I haven't seen this number on the scale since before the kids were born! Every woman, I am sure, can relate.

Then I also begin to think of surgery, recovery, wound healing, and so on; I probably shouldn't lose any more weight. I make myself eat protein bars and drink protein shakes. I choose healthier options than I normally would at restaurants—more fish, vegetables, whole grains. I choose quinoa instead of rice at my lunch bowl spot for the added protein. I almost laugh at myself because I am really not a health-food kind of gal. I grew up in small-town Minnesota; my grandparents were dairy farmers. Whole milk, real butter, meat, potatoes, eggs, bacon (actually side pork) were staples growing up. So it is interesting, in a way, to find I savor the southwest black-bean bowl over quinoa. I make a mental note to try more recipes with quinoa at home.

I start to question some of my other health habits. I do enjoy wine with dinner; Paul and I also have the privilege of hearing live music every Friday night at a coffee shop near our home, the Underground Music Cafe. In addition to coffee, two years ago, they started serving beer, hard cider and wine, along with interesting menu items, including artisan cheese trays, wood-fired pizzas, and the like. We've found our personal favorites that we will sample while listening to a jazz quartet. However, after the breast cancer diagnosis and reading the medical literature, now I can't help but think, *Did I impose some of this upon myself?*

Bottom line: for every alcoholic beverage consumed per day on average, a woman's risk of breast cancer increases by around 8 percent. Even worse, in my opinion, are the studies suggesting that breast tissue is particularly susceptible to the effects of alcohol between menarche and the first full-term pregnancy, which for me was age thirty-two. When I consider college, medical school, even residency, the typical pattern was "Study hard, work hard, play hard." While it wasn't exactly Animal House, it was certainly not unusual for my classmates and me to go to the pub on the weekends or attend parties hosted by the medical fraternity. And apparently, this age range is a time of unusually high risk.

I wonder why this issue is not more widely discussed. I had no idea at the time that this could be harmful to my health other than always designating a sober driver to get us home safely. Even now, most professionals consider a glass of wine a day to have health benefits. It starts to remind me a bit of the tobacco and lung cancer connection. Maybe it's not that strong, but there are some studies suggesting that it is close, yet we seem to be deluding ourselves just a bit. I've seen bottles of wine, for example, being sold during Breast Cancer Awareness month with a pink ribbon on the label. Ah, the irony. If Big Tobacco was and continues to be a powerful force, I can only imagine the same could be said for the industry promoting alcohol. Not just liquor store sales but restaurants, hotels, resorts—the list goes on.

I am still undecided about how to apply this information to myself personally going forward. The above research almost suggests that whatever risk I took on has probably already happened. On the other hand, I delve into numerous articles that discuss the relationship between alcohol consumption and the risk of *recurrence*. Not quite as clear, more research definitely needed. But in the back of my mind, it seems as though consuming alcohol is a bit like playing with fire.

I discover in the early weeks (much as I "discovered" quinoa) that our coffee shop serves a wide variety of excellent herbal teas, hot or iced. Also something called *kombucha*, some sort of fermented carbonated tea beverage, very interesting. My new favorite flavor is sage pear. And luckily, all these options are not only alcohol-free but caffeine-free, which means I can enjoy them on a Friday evening along with the jazz and not be up all night (on top of my newfound insomnia). I start thinking, you know, I could get used to this. Maybe I revert to having wine only on weekends or a special occasion. If there is one thing I've learned in the past few weeks, it's being open to change and trying new things.

Even kombucha.

Chapter 7

THE MENTOR (PART I)

As iron sharpens iron,
so one person sharpens another.
—Proverbs 27:17

As I prepare myself mentally and physically, I am also trying to decide who needs to know about my new diagnosis. I contemplate my circles of friends, family, and colleagues. I try and think about it from the reverse direction: would I be offended if one of them had something like this going on and held it back from me? I have female friends that I would call my circle of trust, women I know either from church, my kid's school, or choir. Telling them, of course, was quite easy for me.

It's work that seems more of a challenge to sort out. I need to tell my division director, Dr. Brad Benson, to sign off on my medical leave paperwork. I am told to notify my clinic medical director, Dr. Lynne Fiscus, to approve the time out of clinic. And of course, I tell my nurse Tony, who is my right-hand man and basically runs the show when I am out of clinic—or even when I am there. Beyond that, well, I am just not sure. For some reason, I am being a bit protective of this new information. I don't want my colleagues to see me in this new light, as prideful as it sounds. Instead of keeping up the image of a competent physician, favorite preceptor, effective course director, active contributor at M&M, advocate for primary care, teacher of students and residents, would it change to "Oh, it's that poor woman who's battling cancer"? I realize I'm worried about somehow being perceived as weak. Irrational, I know, but a concern, nonetheless. And I have the hardest time responding to the simplest greeting in the hallway. One of the GI docs will say, "Hey, Heather! How have you been?" And I'll think, *Hi! I've got cancer! How are you?*

Recently, the U has been placing a lot of emphasis on mentoring. Having been in some formal and informal mentoring relationships over the years, I have found that the informal ones seem to work best; true mentorship has to be unscripted. It is something that naturally falls into place because of mutual shared interests, some commonalities in worldview, respect for the other person's insights and input, and of course, those shared experiences that truly cement the relationship. Physical proximity also plays a huge role; you'd be surprised at how much influence having an office nearby or being assigned adjacent space in clinic really does have. I'd have to say one of those informal mentors for me was Dr. Charles Moldow.

Charlie and I began having these types of interactions many years ago; I'm not even sure when exactly the relationship started, but looking back, he's the type of physician I always aspired to be. A true academician, equally at home teaching students or in a research lab or in high-level leadership roles or seeing patients. He's been the chief of medicine at the VA, an associate dean for research at the medical school. And unlike some in academic medicine—mostly in the younger set, if I dare say so—he did not view teaching or research or administration as a get-out-of-jail-free card, an excuse to shirk away from any and all patient-care responsibilities. He considered patients as not just the one arm of the triple threat but really the center, and it's why we do everything else.

He also has a wicked sense of humor. I appreciated that almost more than anything. In an era when gallows humor was now thought of as politically incorrect; when physicians are not allowed to vent to each other or practice a bit of self-preservation because that wasn't being "patient-centered"; when administrators who never see patients increasingly dictate how, what, when, where we practice; and when we are just expected to go along with it hook, line, and sinker, his candor and humor and incredible insight were like a breath of fresh air.

A few selected Charlie-isms:

On the lack of control over our schedules in primary care: "A person could phone the call center, say they wanted to murder a physician, and they would respond, 'Dr. Thompson has a one-twenty available. Does that work?'"

On the tepid midlevel leadership: "Administration could ask them all to sing the 'Star-Spangled Banner' in the nude, and it would appear as agenda item number 2 at the next monthly meeting."

On the lack of organization of the small-group teaching we both facilitate: "They can't even get the room assignments straight. We are wandering around the entire Academic Health Center like the Jews in the desert."

On the increasing levels of regulation, bureaucracy, and pointless busywork that falls on primary care: "I just spent half an hour doing a preop for an upper endoscopy. Pretty soon, a patient will need a preop to get a haircut."

Charlie has helped me write grants and has read through manuscripts I've drafted for submission; he has written letters of recommendations for me for teaching awards, promotion, and the like. He's also one of the few colleagues who, when I ask him a question or seek his advice, gives an honest, unfiltered opinion without a spin or a slant or caving in to the usual politics of academia. The other point I'd like to mention is that after a few health concerns surfaced for his lovely wife, Gay, he recommended me to be her primary-care doctor. There is no higher honor than this—to have earned the trust and respect of an esteemed colleague to the point of taking care of their spouse. This means more to me than promotion and tenure.

Given all this, I thought, *Well, he should know. He would want to know.* Also, quite frankly, I want his perspective and to benefit from his wisdom, experience, and yes, his sense of humor. But at this point, he's semiretired; he still helps out in resident clinic and with student teaching, but he doesn't have a patient panel of his own. So I have to fill him in via e-mail, not knowing exactly when I will see him next.

I start the e-mail with "Enjoying retirement thus far? We all miss you!" and things of that nature. Then drop the bomb: "I've been diagnosed with breast cancer. Sure is strange to walk into the CSC as a patient, not a doctor."

The reply is only one sentence in length with typos. I happen to know Charlie's a hunt-and-peck typist. Good lord, the EMR must have been torture for him the past several years.

"I woild do ANYTHING for you, just ask." I smile. I breathe a sigh of relief. Then over the coming weeks, he e-mails me about every three days, with his usual thoughtfulness, advice, and yes, wicked sense of humor.

Two days after the first e-mail: "I'm still thinking about you and this diagnosis, the anxiety it must be causing. I can cover your small-group teaching if you need time off."

Advice on breaking the news to my kids: "Tell them one thing at a time. First surgery, then the next steps. Let them ask the questions. They will surprise you." (Which they did.)

Joking about the pending genetic testing and the fact that I don't know my biological father: "You could be half Jewish. Welcome to the community!"

It's a source of encouragement that means so very much to me. I am glad I swallowed my pride and let him in on the full story. Early on, he's only one of two colleagues at the university whom I initially disclose this information to other than a need-to-know basis.

As it turns out, it would have even more meaning down the road.

Chapter 8

Meeting the Surgeon

A trained surgeon knows how to do it; an educated
surgeon knows why we do it. The decision is more
important than the incision.

T hey say that a patient only remembers about 50 percent of
what is told of them during an office visit with a doctor.
Now, experiencing more of this for myself, I say it's
probably even less than that. And this is coming from someone
who *understands* the medical speak. I also find myself having inner
dialogues, things I am thinking to myself but not saying. So here
it is, through the mist and fog of anxiety and uncertainty (coupled
with a somewhat-dangerous baseline medical knowledge), my
recollection of my first meeting with Dr. Todd Tuttle.

He graciously offers me a 7:30 a.m. appointment the very next
day after I sent that staff message, and here I am already fearing I
will be late for it. Surgeons always start their day early; I have two
kids to get up and out of the house for school, and that is always
what holds me up. Anyway, I drove like a bat out of Hades to get
to my parking ramp and then speed-walk to the new Clinics and
Surgery Center (CSC) to the second floor for my appointment.

I have even temporarily forgotten that there is this new
tablet-device-driven electronic check-in process and that as a new
patient, I was supposed to have logged in online and done this
myself the night before. Needless to say, that didn't happen. I get

handed the tablet device, and next thing, I am clicking through a bunch of information. I must click/enter my medical history (hypertension), my family history (same), my medication list (candesartan), my allergies (penicillin), and then "social history": Do I get any exercise? Smoke? Have sex? With whom? Drink alcohol? Chew gum? Shop at Target or Walmart? Mac or PC? Next, the laundry list of symptom questions, and I mean *extensive* list. This is the longest, most torturous check-in I have ever seen.

I am frantically clicking through the review of systems (no, no, no, *no*) when I see Dr. Tuttle casually walking through the lobby. He doesn't seem rushed, but he does stop by the check-in podium and asks the clinic coordinator, "Has my patient arrived yet?" I'm only a few feet away from him in this new "open lobby, no front desk, collaboration zone, touchdown space, flexible workstation" ultramodern building. (My husband tells me, this is all architect-speak for not enough square footage.) I give a little wave, and I say, "I'm here, I'm just checking in!" He looks over, nods, and smiles. It is only five minutes after the appointment time, which is great, for me, in my opinion; but he's in surgical scrubs and clogs. I am probably holding up his first case of the morning and delaying surgery for some poor soul in the fifth-floor operating suite. I feel terrible.

So after the dreaded tablet device, I get a locator badge clipped to my sweater so that the staff can track me down; I feel a bit like a stray dog being chipped at the Humane Society. I am then told to hang out around clinic 2B. There are no designated waiting rooms; I also see there are no magazines or reading materials anywhere, something I hadn't even noticed while practicing in this same building for the past month or so. I think it feels odd, a bit sterile. I like going to my dentist because he has such a great selection for my interests: *Food & Wine, Bon Appétit.* I guess everything here is supposed to be high tech, electronic; I am left with nothing but my phone to entertain me for a few minutes. I check e-mail until I am moved to the station where the nurse takes the vital signs.

After I am in the exam room, it's just a minute and a knock, and in walks Dr. Tuttle. My first impression is that he seems so very calm, so relaxed; maybe it's the scrubs and the clogs, which in my opinion make everyone look a bit like either a tired intern on call or an adult in kid's pajamas. Somehow that feels more approachable to me, or it's just in my wheelhouse or something. He is wearing clear-rimmed glasses and has blond hair with a few streaks of gray, friendly green eyes, and an easy, affable smile. He looks a little bit older than his photo on the UMP website, and that is true, I swear, of every physician I have ever met—including my OB back in the day, the pediatrician for my kids, and my husband's internist. It's as if they take a professional photo of you on the day you start practice, and whether it's been two years or ten years or fifteen, it's the same stock photo they keep posting everywhere. But when meeting him, I actually appreciate seeing those few gray hairs and a touch of a wrinkle. Believe me, in my surgeon, I *want* age, experience, wisdom, opportunity, a lengthy case log—all those things that only come with time.

So I thank him for seeing me and shake his hand; next, I start telling the story: I am reading a book, sitting up in bed, late at night, when I reach down to scratch my chest and I feel this lump beneath the surface of my right breast. I have done self-exams, I mention to him, and this felt different. *In fact, this is the part I didn't tell him: After I went to sleep, I woke up in the morning and thought it might have been a bad dream, so I got in the shower and checked again in the shower. (Wet skin always assists the ability to perform the exam.) At that point, checking the same area, I felt a sinking feeling. Oh no, this is not a dream after all.* I go on to tell him the next steps that led to the cancer diagnosis: the suspicious mammogram, the ultrasound-guided biopsy, the preliminary pathology.

I stop. I think this is probably boring him to death. Surely, he already has seen the images and the path reports; he likely knows all of this.

He then tilts his head slightly, smiles warmly, and asks, "But how are *you* doing?" Inwardly, I think, *Huh, maybe these surgeons are not as brusque as I recall during med school and residency.* My very first clinical rotation as a third-year medical student was surgery at the VA. I had opted for four weeks of general surgery, one week of cardiothoracic surgery, and one week of vascular surgery. There was one general surgeon in particular who was known to eat medical students for breakfast. Lucky for me, I got to scrub in with him on an emergent case, a colonic perforation in an elderly man with either diverticulitis or colon cancer. It was scary as hell, to begin with, and his temper definitely matched. He chewed me out for just about every move I made in the OR; at one point, he rapped me on the knuckles with a hemostat. Later the patient died, not on the table but in the SICU, which threw him into a bad mood for the entire rotation—or maybe that was just his baseline. Some of my experiences on cardiothoracic surgery involved holding retractors and even manually elevating the heart while ice-cold cardioplegia ran over my gloved hand—*for hours.* The vascular surgery people were nice but rounded so darn early; I had to get there by 4:30 a.m. to "pre-round" on my patients prior to 5:30 a.m. chief rounds and 7:00 a.m. cases. I thought, *How can people do this every day?*

Anyway, I am a bit taken aback by his question, not sure how to respond. I say, "I do quite well here during the day. Work is actually a very good thing for me. At night, I have a hard time sleeping; that's when it is more difficult." He smiles. I think for a second he knows exactly what I am talking about. No matter what the situation, physicians tend to throw themselves into their work; it is definitely part of our persona in any specialty. "Physically, I feel fine. I have no pain or any other symptoms. I ran three miles yesterday."

"That's good!" he says, as he gets out a small yellow legal pad and begins to write. "Here is what we know, here is what we don't know, and potential plans going forward." He makes little columns: surgery, chemotherapy, endocrine therapy, mastectomy versus lumpectomy, ER/PR positive versus negative, and so on. He discusses various surgical techniques; he mentions I have two foci in the right breast. With that wide of a margin, we are probably looking not at a lumpectomy but mastectomy plus/minus reconstruction; then he pauses and turns to look at me.

"Reconstruction," I say. "Not sure about that. Tissue expanders, multiple procedures, I just don't know . . ." my voice trails off.

He says firmly: "You really have to be committed to it."

I'm thinking, *Thank you for saying that. That's all I need to know. Reconstruction is not for me.* But I don't say this out loud; I simply nod.

"There's also something known as a nipple-sparing mastectomy, but it's a much fussier procedure."

I think, *Hmm, translate, obviously not for the faint of heart. If an experienced surgeon says this, then I am not going down that road either.* But again, I just nod. He then says, almost thinking out loud, in a moment of . . . frustration? If only it were just the one, not two, how easy this would be.

I ask him if he has many patients who opt not to reconstruct. After doing my research, I realize I am probably in the minority on that one. He says, "If you survey patients down the road, they are equally satisfied whether they choose reconstruction or not." I like that response. The conversation shifts to bilateral: "There is no cancer benefit to undergoing a contralateral prophylactic mastectomy based on what we know about you so far." Ah, good, there's some of that evidence-based medicine and years of outcomes research talking. I am glad he's being so rational about this because, despite my best efforts, I feel emotions creeping in left and right. At first, I think, *Spare the left!* At least I can keep the good one! Then I hear later about some ill-defined area of enhancement in the left breast on imaging, and I think, *Hack them both off! Tomorrow!*

This is probably why Dr. Tuttle has the calmest bedside demeanor I think I've ever seen in a practitioner other than perhaps Sam's first pediatrician, who was on the verge of retirement and barely had a pulse. I would cultivate that, too, if I were dealing every single day with stressed patients who just learned of a new cancer diagnosis and had to make decisions that potentially affect them for their entire lives in just a span of a few days to a few weeks. You certainly would have to call upon your own endogenous cannabinoids to counteract the adrenaline effects radiating from the person sitting in the opposite chair.

Because there are still quite a few tests pending—including an MRI ordered by my primary MD, special stains for ER, PR, HER2—we actually don't have that much more to talk about. He does think I should seek genetic testing, including an appointment with a genetic counselor. He mentions I should see Anne Blaes. I think, *Well, you must be right. You are the third physician, including myself, to spontaneously recommend her.* He offers a referral to a plastic surgeon. Inwardly, I think, *Thanks, but that is not going to be necessary.* Nearing the end of the visit, he writes down a number on the yellow legal paper and says, "Call me anytime. This is my cell phone." He then slides the piece of paper over toward me. I quickly grab it and place it in my purse; I will refer to this later, multiple times actually, to help me remember the details we discussed—the other 50 percent.

I thank him, this time out loud, and then I mention that his cell phone could also be his pager. "What?" I tell him about page copy, a service available to all physicians in our group practice where your pages are automatically forwarded to your cell phone as a text message, essentially rendering the pager obsolete. Carry one device, not two, which is great especially on the weekends. "How come I didn't know about this?" he says with a laugh. Now suddenly we're on common ground. So we spend the last few minutes commiserating about the new building we are sitting in.

"How do you like the new building?" I ask, probably with a slight smirk on my face. Line up ten of our physicians and ask them this question, and you will get a startling range of answers. There is a shuttle service from the hospital to the new clinic building; if the shuttle is full of only MDs, they immediately start comparing notes about how their clinic is operating in the new space compared to the old. They really should bug that shuttle if they want any feedback on how to improve. "Oh, the *building*, why, of course, the building itself is very nice." Now it is he who has a smirk on his face. "But all of this . . ." He gestures first to my high-tech locator badge, then circles his finger in the air to indicate the entirety of it. "Well, *this* needs a lot of work going forward."

Now that is yet another thing we already agree upon.

Chapter 9

Meeting (Again) the Oncologist

Oncologists and their patients are bound, it seems, by
an intense subatomic force.
—Siddhartha Mukherjee, The Emperor of All Maladies

Before my appointment had even ended with Dr. Tuttle, I
had been scheduled a second appointment two days later
with Dr. Anne Blaes. This one was on a Friday morning,
and I usually have clinic of my own all day Friday. I needed to
have one of our nurses reschedule several early morning patients,
with short notice and no offer of any explanation. As mentioned
earlier, I haven't decided yet how I want to disclose my diagnosis
at work or who needs to know. Usually, I tend to be a rather-
private person, yet here I am in my own clinic building, seeking
care for a new, life-changing, long-term medical condition. And
of course, when I had wandered through the second floor, looking
for the check-in podium for Dr. Tuttle's appointment, one of the
coordinators said jokingly, "Dr. Thompson, are you lost? Your
clinic is on the fourth floor!" (Remember, we've only been in this
new building about four weeks, so I actually could have been
lost.) I also saw a patient of mine whom I know very well walking
through the clinic 2B area; she stared for a bit as I was sitting in a
lounge chair, maybe not quite recognizing me without the white
coat and stethoscope.

So this really is a juxtaposition of my internal values, my personality profile (INFJ, if interested) versus my desire to have the very best people involved in my care. I wanted to draft the A team, and to do that, I had to set aside these preconceived notions of how I must separate work from my personal life. It's really a bit of a joke, anyway; those lines have become more and more blurred over the years in different ways, especially with the advent of technology, including the EMR. I do almost as much work from home as at the office because I can access my patient's charts from anywhere. At first, I resented this; now I embrace it because it gets me home at a decent hour, and that's what my kids notice most.

So here I am again, doing the dance for a second time. The appointment is at 8:30 a.m. A little after 8:00 a.m., I am walking through the front lobby of my hospital in order to catch that shuttle that goes over to the new clinic building. I am looking around, watching doctors and nurses, as well as patients, streaming in and out through the revolving doors, everyone in a hurry, off to something important, when I see Dr. Anne Blaes also walking through the lobby at a fast clip, looking down at her phone. Funny, I think, here we are both rushing off to the exact same appointment. I could see in the EMR that I'm the first patient scheduled for her. I hang back and let her pass me for some reason. I wonder if she already saw me. I wonder if she will walk or ride the shuttle; I will do the opposite. I'm trying not to impose or invade her personal/professional space any more than I will need to in the coming hours (days, weeks, months). It's a nice morning, and the sun is shining, so I decide to walk, either way.

This time, check-in is faster. I don't have to fill out the lengthy tablet health history, thank God, and I am ushered quickly into the vital-signs area. My blood pressure is not too bad. I must be a bit less anxious this time. I have begun to process the situation, and that's good. Or maybe it was just that awful tablet device.

A knock and into the room enters Dr. Blaes. She's quite tall, with shoulder-length, straight ash-blonde hair. She has an angular jaw and very pale-blue eyes. She's wearing a gray sweater over black pants under the requisite white coat. I've known her for many years, and unlike the rest of us, she seems not to age or change one bit. Those ice-blue eyes can be a bit intimidating;

I've thought this before as we've met and discussed, for example, student concerns about the course we were codirecting. Her communication style tends to be very direct, matter of fact, to the point; I would not say warm or fuzzy. I had often wondered, in our teaching roles, how she comes across to a student who is begging for additional attendance points because their dog was sick or their sister had gallbladder surgery or their husband was being sworn in at the bar or the myriad of other reasons we hear to turn an "unexcused" absence into an "excused" for more points. Not that she is unsympathetic. Fair, ethical, holds everyone to a very high standard—that is how I would describe her with students. Her patients would describe her as a fierce advocate, a physician who always goes the extra mile. I am okay with all of this, and I don't really need warm fuzzy as long as I am getting the most accurate, evidence-based information.

She extends her hand. "I'm sorry we have to be meeting this way!" she begins. Yes, indeed, I agree but thank her for seeing me. "Tell me how this came about, and tell me about your overall health." I detail the events leading up to the diagnosis in a similar fashion to Dr. Tuttle's appointment. I mention the blood pressure. I tell her I feel great, no symptoms, still running for exercise, trying to give her the whole picture because I know as well as she does that functional status matters in terms of outcomes.

She gets out a piece of paper that is a fax from the outside care system; it's my biopsy report. On the left side are the standard descriptors—histologic type, histologic grade, and so on. On the right side, she begins a column jotting down her interpretation of all this. Technically, there are two tumors, two primaries, both about one centimeter in size, both stage T1bN0 so far. They are both ER/PR positive, we now know; HER2 FISH is pending. Her columns start to mimic very much the ones written by Dr. Tuttle: surgery, radiation, chemotherapy, endocrine therapy. Her first point: "At stage 1, your treatment is primarily surgical." Her second point: "You are young. We need to consider adjuvant therapy. Once there is a local or distal recurrence, there is not much we can do."

Boom. Those words hung in the air, weighed heavily on my mind, and would echo in the days to come. If there's anything I would remember from this visit, it was that statement. I hadn't really thought that far ahead, to be honest; I was still considering the surgical approach and researching those various aspects. She must have seen the look on my face, and I think I mumbled something like "Well, hopefully, I have a lot of years left." On that note, Dr. Blaes drew a new graph. Something called the Oncotype assay, a test which will be run on the tumor itself (not just a blood test as I had assumed); this is all news to me. With these results returning low, intermediate, or high probability of recurrence, a decision would have to be made regarding chemotherapy.

"What kind of chemotherapy are we talking about?" I ask, knowing there is chemo and then there is *chemo* with a wide range of side effects and toxicities. If HER2 is positive, it's weekly Taxol and Herceptin. If HER2 negative, Docetaxel, and Cytoxan every three weeks for four cycles. Ugh. "Would I be able to work?" is my next question. "Well, now you know Becky . . ." she says with a soft smile. Dr. Marsh's kind face flashes back into my mind; her name is all over the pathology report sitting in front of us. "She is still working. Most patients find that this regimen gives them fatigue on day 4; the steroids help day 1 to 3. If you time it right, those bad days can fall on the weekend."

Weekend? What weekend? I'm doing some work, even at home, every day, certain times more than others. Then it's as though she read my mind: "Do you have any inpatient attending coming up?" These are the weeks when we round daily at the hospital, regardless of weekends or holidays, and we take care of the sickest patients in the Twin Cities. Luckily, it's April; I have only one week assigned in June, and then nothing on the schedule yet going forward since the academic year begins July 1. "I would advise not doing any inpatient attending while on chemo." Then I start to think of more mundane issues: *my hair!* I've had the same stylist, Michelle, since before Sam was born; I'm way overdue for another cut and foil highlights, and now I am thinking, *Why bother if it's all going to fall out?* Again, it's as though she read my mind. "We have this new cooling cap that can prevent hair loss. Basically, it vasoconstricts all the blood vessels in your scalp. Insurance will even cover it." Fine and dandy, I think, but let's just hope it does not come to that.

We move on to the perfunctory physical exam; I tell her I'm leaning toward no reconstruction; I really just want the simplest surgical procedure and whatever gets my life back sooner. She asks me about my kids and hobbies. "Are you still singing in that choir?"

Wow, I think, *I can't believe she remembers that.* It's the Oratorio Society of Minnesota, a community choir that I've been a member of since medical school. I told her ironically I took this semester off because of Sam's basketball games and practice schedules; now in retrospect, that was one less thing on my plate, and I'm thankful. "You can always go back to it, I bet." True enough. She also asks how I am holding up mentally. I tell her about the insomnia, but that half a tablet of Benadryl is my new best friend. "Let me know if you need something more than that."

I thank her, but despite being an internist, I'm a bit of a medication nihilist; no amount of SSRI or benzodiazepine really changes the fact that cancer sucks—even this stage 1 cancer, which I am realizing more and more how blessed I am to have discovered it myself, this early. What are the chances that I would have an itch and scratch just this one area? And while sitting up in bed, propped on pillows, reading, likely enhancing the position of my chest *just so,* in that I easily recognized this was not my usual bumpiness . . . Thinking about that is starting to freak me out a bit. But it also just reinforces my belief that in life, there really are no coincidences.

"I will need to see you back about three weeks post-op." Post-op? Oh, that's right, I will be having surgery. I don't have a date yet; it seems so abstract. I shake her hand as she is about to leave; for a split second, I wanted to hug her, and I am not really sure why. I catch myself smile and nod. Remember, no warm fuzzy. I get off the exam table, put back on my clothes, and in fifteen minutes, I'm seeing my first patient two floors above.

Chapter 10

THE MRI SAGA

I've been looking so long at these pictures of you, that I
almost believe that they're real.
—The Cure

You haven't really lived until you have experienced the
MRI machine. It is quite amazing, this technology and
the beautifully detailed images it produces; but the entire
process, well, it's just humorous at best, frightening at worst. I can
see why some patients panic and have to be pulled out of the tube.
And now, I can also appreciate the difficulties in interpreting the
results.

My first MRI was at Regions Hospital in St. Paul. The
abnormal mammogram and ultrasound were followed
immediately by a core biopsy on the right side. I then get the
call, 8:00 a.m. on the following Tuesday, that the biopsies were
positive for two different cancers, two different types, each less
than two centimeters, about two centimeters apart from one
another. (Rule of 2?) This was picked up almost incidentally by
the astute radiologist via ultrasound; I thought I had detected by
self-exam only one. Because the finding was rather surprising to
my primary MD (although, later, Dr. Blaes commented that she's
seen this before), an MRI was ordered to better detail both the
right and left breast. I called around, and Regions was the only
place to offer me the first available appointment that very same

day, and so that is why I chose to drive halfway across town in rush-hour traffic. And technically, I had not yet been referred to the university, or I could have probably had it done right there in my own building.

The appointment was scheduled at 6:45 p.m., and they told me to expect about an hour to complete the exam. I was a bit disappointed because that meant I wouldn't get home until 8:00 p.m., and that is nearing my kids' bedtime. At this point, I had not told them the news yet, so I didn't really want to explain the real reason why I was getting home so late. (I guess I could always tell them I was waiting on an MRI. They've heard that one before!) And looking at my schedule, it made sense. I had my own patients until 5:00 p.m.; therefore, I could assume I would be finished by 6:00 p.m. and not be late.

So imagine my surprise when I get a call on my cell phone from Regions at around 4:00 p.m.: "We've had an unexpected cancellation. Can you come at five o'clock?" I was about to say no when I pulled up my schedule in the EMR and . . . *the last two patients had dropped off my schedule.* The 4:00 p.m. and 4:30 p.m. appointment slots sat empty with a "green square" right next to them (meaning, they are a go, and they could be filled at any minute). *What are the chances?* I walk over to my medical assistant with my phone still held to my ear. "Can you block those last two appointments?" I say to her, again with no explanation. She just nods wordlessly and turns to the computer to make it so. "Yes, I can be there at 5:00 p.m.! Thanks for calling!" I say into the phone. I disconnect, pause, and look heavenward for a second; and after thanking God for that small miracle, I head to the locker room to hang up my white coat, grab my purse, and leave.

It is still rush hour, however, and 94 East is stop-and-go the entire way. I had just enough time to get to the patient visitor ramp by about 4:50 p.m. Now, the funny thing is, my residency program rotated through three hospitals: the VA, the university, and you guessed it, Regions. So taking the exit off the freeway and turning onto Roberts Street felt very familiar even if it was so many years ago. I also vaguely remembered where the MRI scanner was. Basement, of course, always in the basement, and it was right down the hall from some sort of physical-therapy pool. It smelled like chlorine as you were getting closer, and so once again, after all this time, it was that familiar chlorine odor that let me know I was headed in the right direction in the lower-level maze of hallways and doors.

I present at the front desk for check-in. A wristband is placed, and I am ushered into a locker room, where I change into scrubs. Two very nice RNs greet me once I am out; they are going through a standard checklist (no, I don't have any shrapnel in my body) and then start an IV. Next, I am led over to the actual MRI scanner, and I see this contraption that looks like a doughnut, where you would place your head facedown, for example, while getting a nice upper-body massage at the mall or at the airport. Only, unlike the mall, there are two square cutouts right below that, one for each breast, and two armrests at either side, on the end of this long cart on wheels designed to move you in and out of the machine. It's also about four feet off the floor, and I see a tiny step stool leading up to it; I am thinking, you would have to have the agility of a gymnast to navigate this without any help! How do eighty-year-old ladies do it?

I get to put on a surgical bouffant to keep my shoulder-length hair from getting in the way. Next, somehow I manage to climb up into this thing and position myself adequately, knowing I want to be comfortable enough not to move around for quite some time to avoid creating any distortion of the images. That is no easy task because, despite the foam cushioning, it feels a bit like I am lying facedown on a very hard plastic lawn chair with my chest protruding between two of the slats.

They give me headphones and select my choice of music. Thank God for that; it was a welcome distraction. I am wheeled in, and I ask them to crank the volume up. Despite this, when the MRI machine starts up, I nearly jump out of my skin. *It is so loud!* And it has this very strange sound quality to it, like the constant wail of discordant bagpipes that are playing right next to your head. Throughout the exam, this sound would start and stop, stuttering at times, and then change pitch. I'd think, here come the T2 weighted images. I am holding perfectly still, my right hand around that panic button but not pressing it. I am taking the smallest, most shallow guppy breaths through my mouth with barely parted lips. I do not want "Image quality limited by motion artifact" on my report, thank you very much.

It seems like an eternity, but the scan is finally over. I breathe a sigh of relief as I am wheeled out of the machine. "You did great!" they all say. I think, *Well, you do what you have to do to get answers.* But I am glad they seem so confident because these images may help inform the next steps.

Fast-forward: The MRI report comes back showing again the two areas on the right, but then also commenting on an area of enhancement on the left breast, superior aspect. My first highly irrational thought: I am simply riddled with cancer. Why not schedule a bilateral mastectomy *right now* and just be done with it? Even in a panic moment, I send a text message to Dr. Tuttle saying basically just that.

His reply: "Premature. If this little thing in your left breast is cancer, I want to know it before surgery." He instead recommends getting a second look ultrasound and possibly a biopsy on that left side.

Ah, well, yes, I suppose. The man's right; I am jumping to premature conclusions. I remind myself: I chose this surgeon for this very reason, because of his thought process and evidence-based surgical decision-making. But wow, was it hard to remember that in the early weeks? In these crazy moments, when I found myself doubting and, yes, panicking, I had to remind myself time and again to *just give in, trust, and follow his lead.* Rereading his text, I begin to calm down a bit. And in fact, over the next few days, I start to think about that left breast a lot, and eventually, I start to form my own ideas.

Thinking more about this, I have always had fairly predictable breast pain the week before my cycle. More so on the left side. In fact, it's how I would be alerted to the upcoming fun. I would get really mad if the left breast hurt, for example, the week before a planned vacation. In my years of self-exams, I also thought I had felt much more "lumpy, bumpy" tissue on the left compared to the right; putting that together with the pain, I reasoned I had fibrocystic change.

I realize in the coming days that the first MRI was done right before the start of my cycle. Huh, that little flash of contrast was probably just hormonally active tissue. I have been checking, *daily even,* that left breast for any lumps; there is nothing there that I have not felt before. I start to think, *They aren't going to find anything on that ultrasound*, which is exactly what happens.

I am scheduled for the ultrasound at noon on a Wednesday, one week following Dr. Tuttle's appointment. I get to meet our own breast-imaging team, Dr. Tim Emory and his fellow, Brian. They are great, so respectful; they keep addressing me as Dr. Thompson, which sounds strange, but I stop correcting them. They press in, they probe, and they hem and haw but can't find anything to biopsy. Still not satisfied, they recommend proceeding with an MRI-directed biopsy of this supposed area of enhancement on the left. Even though I have my doubts, I say, "Okay, when do you want me back?" They schedule me for the following Tuesday morning, which is the only day they perform these MRI-directed breast biopsies. Providentially again, it works for me. My schedule is open until 1:00 p.m., but I am a little disappointed; it's another week of waiting, which for me is excruciating.

That morning, April 12, I get up, and I am leaving the house around 7:30 a.m. for the 8:30 a.m. appointment in radiology. I grab my phone off the charger, and I see a text: "Good luck with your biopsy! Let's talk when we get the final results!" I read it, and I think, who *is* this? My mom? My friend Jodie? It's a 612 number that I don't immediately recognize, and it doesn't have a name attached in my contacts. Then I read it through again, and I realize that it's my surgeon, Dr. Todd Tuttle.

Now, if I ever had any doubts that I had a fantastic team pulling for me in every way, those were immediately erased by seeing that text. The impact of that one simple text cannot be underestimated. It wasn't just the medical knowledge or the technical expertise but also the moral support that truly amazed me. It also showed me that everyone else was paying attention, waiting on these results; it was not just me having to sweat it out alone in this state of mind. I again thought of the radiologist and her excellent advice to seek care at the U, and I cannot imagine that I ever even contemplated going anywhere else. I am going to bleed maroon and gold on that operating table.

So I text back, "Thank you! Sounds great!" And I hop in the car, drive on into the brand-new Clinics and Surgery Center, heading over to first-floor radiology. But I'm totally convinced by now that there is nothing on the left side and this is an exercise in futility. I feel like placing bets with the radiologist just for fun.

I'm becoming a pro at this by now—the routine, the changing into scrubs, the IV, the "any metal in your body" questionnaire. I am led into the MRI suite, and it is brand new, stark white, high ceilings, more modern than Regions but less welcoming, less cozy, if you can actually describe a radiology suite that way. I check out the doughnut-hole contraption once again. This time, the right-sided opening below it is covered up. Just the left one remains.

I recognize the fellow Brian, who comes in with a new attending radiologist. She shakes my hand. *"You're* Dr. Heather Thompson! I see your name all the time on orders." She's standing there with a typical teaching entourage, including the fellow, two students. We're all smiling at each other as if this is meeting over coffee or at the water cooler. Again, the expression of "I'm sorry we have to meet this way" comes up, and several heads nod. I am just looking at all of them, taking it in. Brian starts to describe the entire process to me (part of the informed consent, I realize), and I let him explain to me in detail how they perform the actual biopsy while I am in and out of the MRI scanner. It sounds so very strange even to me and quite complicated the way the machine has to be exactly lined up in the correct space and whatnot. I don't like the sounds of it.

Finally, he stops. Everyone is now looking at me. "Any questions?"

"No," I say, but this time, I decide to go out on a limb. "But I don't think you are going to find anything there. This area on my left breast that you are interested in—I have felt some bumpiness there before, for many years, and always a bit of tenderness right before my cycle, and that was the unfortunate timing of the MRI last week. I know you have to take a look, but that's my opinion."

They just nod and say, "Well, let's see." No one offers to place a bet.

So up and in I go; this machine has one distinct disadvantage— it's so new that the foam cushioning is a bit stiff, and it's actually even less comfortable (if that is possible) than the MRI at Regions. And unfortunately, this time it is even more important that I don't move around based on that above description of events. On the other hand, once it fires up, I notice it is not quite as loud as the scanner last week. Maybe newer technology has been able to dampen the noise or something to that effect.

But at least I have the headphones and music again with another distinct difference: the radio service offered at Regions was commercial-free; here, they must have opted for the less-expensive version because pretty soon, I'm hearing about Dave's Carpet Cleaning while the bagpipes wail in the background. I laugh, inwardly of course—guppy breaths.

After a bit, the wailing stops. I hear through the microphone speaker: "Doing okay?"

"Yep!" I say.

"We'll just be reviewing this for a bit."

Time passes. Suddenly, I am abruptly wheeled out of the machine. I lift my head and rest my chin on the doughnut. Brian comes around to the front of the table and stoops a bit so his face is at my eye level. "We didn't see anything light up on the images, so we are not going to biopsy."

"I told you so!" I said with a big smile. If there is one thing I know, it's that doctors really enjoy being right.

He starts laughing. Actually, all four of them are laughing now—the radiologist, the fellow, and the two students. It's a joyful noise, hearing that warm laughter echo through the cold MRI suite, so I join in.

A very old quote comes to mind from Henry Ward Beecher. "Mirth is God's medicine. Everybody ought to bathe in it." I'm starting to agree. I feel a huge release, a palpable lightening of the heavy load, with all of us cracking up. I'm bathing in it.

And *kind of a big deal*—the left one can stay. I am very pleased. It was always the better of the two, anyway.

While I was relieved to hear this, in retrospect, I am not entirely sure I needed that first MRI to begin with. As I reflect on it, it is very telling how one abnormal result initially leads to panic, then from one additional test to another, yet just as we were taught in medical school, ultimately, the scan must be interpreted in the clinical context. My own symptoms and exam were still relevant, a powerful reminder of how the history and physical together with evidence-based medicine can inform our practice and reduce unnecessary testing. It could save not only health-care dollars but time and energy spent in follow-up, as well as the anxiety surrounding it.

And hopefully, avoid another MRI saga.

Chapter 11

THE SURGERY DATE

Just one question, I might ask ya,
And it might sound like a disaster,
But can you make this thing . . . go . . . faster?
—The Black Crowes

Right after the MRI, I send another text to Dr. Tuttle.

"MRI didn't show anything."

"Great! Do you have a moment to talk?" he texts back.

"I'm riding the shuttle. Maybe in five minutes?"

"Sure. Call me when you get the chance."

I get back to my office, and we connect via phone. First I tell him I've decided against reconstruction. I just want a speedy recovery, I say, but also I mention that the waiting is really getting to me. He says, "Yes, let's get the surgery date scheduled." He's presumably looking at a calendar and says, "What about next week? April 20?" Although on some level I'd say yes to *tomorrow*, I do mention that it might be better to look into the week following, or further out, mainly to have fewer patients of my own to reschedule. I also remember I am supposed to attend a ceremony on April 20 for a medical school teaching award, and although it is rather silly (I really didn't need to be there in person), I was sort of looking forward to that as a morale booster. Hearing some accolades, not just for me but for my fellow colleagues, and then socializing at a reception afterward, that sounds like a welcome break from the clinic appointments and MRI scans and everything else I've been having to endure recently.

"Yes, that should work. I will have my scheduler call you back with the exact date and time." I mention I already have a pre-op arranged for April 15. Then I ask him, "Do you think I will be admitted to the hospital?" I'm trying to anticipate how much I will need help with the kids that week. "Knowing you, I would say you will likely go home the same day."

Wow, that would be truly amazing. I've spent enough time, probably *years* of my life, from medical student to resident to attending within in the physical confines of the University of Minnesota Medical Center. To be at home, recovering in my own bed, sounds wonderful to me. When I had my kids, I thought being hospitalized was next to torture even though everything went fine. Lydia arrived at 6:00 a.m. on a Sunday; by 6:00 a.m. on that Monday, I was dressed, all of my things packed up, infant in car seat, when the team tried to round on me. *I am outa here.* In fact, because I was in the hospital less than twenty-four hours, they forgot to draw the newborn screening for metabolic disorders, and I had a public health nurse calling me that very same day in a panic, asking me to report to the nearest laboratory STAT.

So the next step is to really clear my calendar. I'm glad I had already reached out to Charlie; I may need him for last-minute resident clinic coverage. But what about the med students? I have a weekly clinical medicine small group; I also have a student working with me every Tuesday afternoon in clinic. Will I have to arrange different "substitute teachers" for all this? If so, then more people will notice I am gone and might start to ask questions. I decide to pull up the year-long medical school calendar on the website. As it turns out, the week I will have surgery is a final-exam week, and the week following, a late spring break for the students. *No pressing need to make any special arrangements.* The timing incredibly is absolutely perfect.

Then I get a call with the actual date and time: "We have you scheduled for April 26, 10:00 a.m. You will need to report to 3C by 8:00 a.m." Ironically, this just happens to be our thirteenth wedding anniversary. I think, *Well, this could be a real downer. Cancel those Chianti Grill dinner reservations.* But for some reason, I didn't ask to change the date. I think I just wanted to get it over and done with. And eventually, rather than feel disappointed, I decide to view it as a positive thing. It's going to be a brand-new anniversary from now on, celebrating *two things*—both the wedding date, and anniversary of being cancer-free. God willing.

And same as it was securing that first appointment with Dr. Tuttle, just having the surgery date set, for some reason, is a real source of comfort. I would stare at it, contemplating the future on my Google Calendar. I'd see it, looming ahead, whenever I would log into the EMR and look at my own clinic schedule by calendar date. But up until the actual day of surgery, I wasn't nervous or worried about it, just more anticipating—wanting to move forward, feeling the need to jump and clear that first hurdle. In some ways, as I look back, April 12 to April 26 was the longest two weeks of my life.

I also began to contemplate ways to apply this in my own practice. Come to think of it—I already do on a much smaller scale. I have a handful of patients, probably only five to six, that I see every month in clinic regardless of what is going on, because just having that appointment seems to help. Tony knows exactly who they are. Having those scheduled visits with me (even if I only check their blood pressure or repeat one basic lab or refill their medication), well, it keeps them out of the ER, and that is huge. Once, when I was out on my second maternity leave, one of these patients—who had been sober for years—went out on a binge-drinking episode, developed acute pancreatitis with prolonged hospitalization, drainage of a fluid collection, on and on. After my return, I told her I was done having kids, and I scheduled her back every four weeks . . . to this day.

But it's not just those "needy" patients who deserve this. Here I am, a well-educated, medically trained individual, relatively high functioning (most days); and I could feel a tangible lowering of my anxiety level with these incredibly simple interventions. I decide I am no longer going to leave my patients unless they are completely healthy with open-ended follow-up. I'm bringing them back, maybe not all of them in four weeks (huge backlog potential!) but in two months, three months, six months. I'll request that the clinic coordinators actually *give* them an appointment date and time on their way out rather than just handing them the number to the call center. I think I might have a new appreciation for what it means to provide patient-centered care, none of which are standard items on the Press Ganey. But I'm going to try it, nonetheless.

Chapter 12

THE OR

When undergoing surgery, console yourself with the
reflection that you are giving the doctor pleasure and
he is getting paid for it.
—Mark Twain

General anesthesia is so weird. You go to sleep in one
room, wake up in a totally different room four hours
later. Just like in college.
—Ross Schafer

The morning of the surgery, I have to take a shower with this specialized antibacterial skin soap that smells absolutely terrible. It actually reminds me of anatomy lab with the pervasive scent of formaldehyde that enters every strand of hair, every pore in your skin, every layer of clothing you could possibly wear. I'm also terribly nervous. Why, I am not sure; I know I am in great hands. I have every confidence in Dr. Tuttle's skill, and ever since having an epidural for both deliveries, I think anesthesiologists walk on water. I've never been so happy to see a doctor walk into a room as I was when I had just entered active labor with Sam. It's a Sunday afternoon, which is probably a good thing—no scheduled cases in the OR. The doc is there about thirty seconds after I yell, "Page anesthesia!" After popping in the catheter, the medication starts to flow; the horrible visceral, gut-wrenching pain dissipates. I go from the wailing and the gnashing of the teeth to actually smiling, and I say to him,

"Thank you! Thank you! Oh my goodness, what a difference!" He turns to me and says in a soft and soothing tone, "I rarely make anything worse," and just silently drifts out of the room like the Lone Ranger. Who was that masked man?

But I suppose nerves get the best of me today, in part because I have seen unexpected, unanticipated outcomes over the years. I've been to a morning report case, a woman who developed acute hepatitis then fulminant hepatic failure, presumably as a reaction to the anesthesia. I think about the bruising that developed in my right breast after the core biopsy, and I wonder if that means anything, any predictor of bleeding complications, such as a hematoma. I help teach the six-week course on hematology; I know about platelet defects and everything else that can interfere with hemostasis. I realize that I am *really* overthinking this, but I can't help it.

So Paul and I report to the perioperative area known as 3C in the hospital at 8:00 a.m. We check in and get to hang out in the patient and family lounge. It's a bit strange, being on the patient side. As a resident and now attending, I've admitted patients who have failed recovery from 3C to the inpatient medicine service; I've scrubbed into these same ORs as a medical student. But I am finding that while, yes, it's a bit surreal, it's also somewhat comforting. It's helping my nerves just a bit. I've been here before; I know where everything is located. Even the hallways and exam rooms and the decor are all very familiar; the same framed prints are still up on the walls, the same privacy curtains hang with their floral pattern. Later, I would stare up at the ceiling and walls in OR 14 and think, *There's that pale-green tile I remember, hasn't changed a bit.*

First things first, I am asked to give a urine sample (gotta make sure I'm not pregnant) and then get completely undressed and into this warming device known as the Bair Hugger. The nurse helps me with it. It's a bit awkward, and she turns up the heat via a dial on the side. I do get to put on these nice dark-green footie socks with the grips on the bottom, but otherwise, you are as naked as the day you came into this world. Even during labor and delivery, I got to keep my cute floral maternity/nursing top nightgown on the entire time, so this feels strange. I decided to keep my contact lenses in and not tell anybody. I was envisioning waking up in the PACU, groggy from anesthesia and not being able to see anything to boot. Besides, I've taken longer naps with my contacts in place and did just fine.

But I knew I was still nervous when the nursing staff had to resort to not one, not two, but *four* attempts to start a peripheral IV in my left arm (and I'm usually an easy stick). I'm a bit dehydrated, NPO, and totally peripherally clamped down from the epinephrine. They finally obtain access, but it takes a while. During this time, I am also meeting the anesthesiologist, Dr. Iannazzo. She's in scrubs, of course, bouffant hat, and mask loosely draped around her neck; but she has this perfectly applied makeup accenting her big blue eyes. Silver eye shadow, gray eyeliner, and black mascara on curled lashes. I look into those lovely eyes and sort of study them, knowing that's all I will see, if I do see any of her face in the OR. She's describing what will happen next; I tell her I'm a bit nervous, and she's saying, "That's understandable. As soon as we get that darn IV in, I can give you medication to relax you." I'm also worried about post-op nausea and vomiting. To me, nausea is almost worse than pain (again, flashback to pregnancy).

"Do you get motion sickness?" she asks.

I tell her, "No, I love roller coasters, love spinning rides."

"Then you'll do fine! Believe me, there's a strong correlation."

After a few more standard instructions, I finally tell her I am an internal medicine doc. "What? Why didn't you tell me sooner? Where do you work?"

"Here," I say.

"Wow! That's great! So you already know all this stuff!" We get to chat a bit more informally now. She tells me she also went to medical school at the University of Minnesota, then onto Mayo for residency. She has two young kids. She says I really need to check out this Facebook organization designed as a support network for female physicians who are also moms. More free advice and life coaching.

Right before that, Dr. Tuttle had stopped in. He's wearing tan pants, a striped button-down shirt, and navy-blue sports coat. I say, "Boy, am I glad to see you. I have something to get off my chest." He tilts his head to the side for a second, looks at me quizzically, not realizing I am trying to crack a joke. Then he gets it and laughs. I am obviously way too nervous; I totally botched the timing and delivery on that one. He seems upbeat as usual but also pauses, looks around the room, and says, "This must be sort of weird for you."

I tell him, "Yes and no."

Next, he marks the surgical site with an X, a patient-safety maneuver for many years now. Then he sits down. I've been lying flat on my back, staring at the ceiling; I'm starting to sweat from the heat blowing through that Bair Hugger device. I roll onto my left side, turn the dial down, and prop up on an elbow so I can be facing him, making eye contact. He starts to rattle off a few instructions: "You are going to be peeing blue for the next twenty-four hours. Showering is okay but no soaking in a tub. No lifting anything greater than ten pounds. Avoid NSAIDs until post-op day 5. You can eat or drink anything you want, later tonight, but no booze." (Yes, he says booze.) I smile and inwardly think, *Well, that one's easy these days.*

His resident enters the room and introduces herself as Dr. Skube. She has long dark hair tied back in a ponytail. She has a baby bump, I'm pretty sure. God bless her. I think having a baby during surgical residency is bold. We have a joke about internal medicine residency post the duty-hour restrictions: The pregnancy rate increased by about 400 percent once we eliminated overnight call. It's either, the married residents have too much time on their hands, turning toward other nocturnal activities, or they are emboldened by the prospect of having slightly more humane hours and some actual free time to spend with their baby and family at home. So while here we thought it would be easier to create the call schedule, just inserting weeks of night float here and there in blocks, we also found a new problem, in that we had to accommodate a bunch of maternity leaves. Interesting, don't you think?

Dr. Skube is now talking about post-op pain medication. She's printing out a prescription for oxycodone, 5 mg tablets. This is about the same time that the nurses are trying to start that IV. As the anesthesiologist enters, she and Dr. Tuttle make a quick exit. I envision both of them going back to change into scrubs and wonder if the locker rooms still look the same, with that machine with the scanner ID card that dispenses the OR scrubs and the racks of shoe covers and hair bouffants and masks. The color of the scrubs changed from teal green to a more standard blue about ten years ago. I still have my vintage green scrubs from my intern year in 1998; they are incredibly soft from now almost two decades of washing, and I still wear them when I do night shifts.

So after the IV is in, all things are go so to speak; a male nurse anesthetist enters the room and says, "Happy hour." I have no idea what he's got, but I assume it's a benzo, and pretty soon I do feel nice and floaty, and I must have a smile or a more relaxed expression on my face because as I'm being wheeled back, he says, "Now that's a much better look for you." Down the hall, past the familiar surroundings, we enter OR 14 with the pale-green tile. I am lifted onto the operating table, and I don't remember anything after that.

Next: hearing voices. "EBL 10 cc. No urine yet." (*Did I get a foley?* I wonder. *Naw, I think the case would be too short.*) Another familiar voice, I think it's Dr. Tuttle: "Heather? Heather? Are you awake?" I'm tired, so incredibly tired. I just want to go back into that deep and dreamless sleep. I opened my eyes for a second; it was him. I can't remember what he said next or if I said anything in return. I hear another voice, perhaps Dr. Iannazzo? "I'm glad she held that ARB. Blood pressure was perfect." I feel myself being moved around a bit, jostled from side to side. I think someone slips the bouffant off my head. A female voice says, "Her hair looks better than mine." People laugh. Soon after, the bedside nurse was talking to me in soothing tones. "Everything went fine." After a few more minutes, I am a bit more awake. It's really a battle, though. I'm trying to force myself to keep my eyes open and shake off this fuzzy sensation.

Ironically, next thing, the same nurse comes back, this time with a syringe of Dilaudid. I sit up a bit more. I think, *But wait, I'm trying to wake up. That's going to snow me!* I say something to that effect; she dials back the dose from 0.5 mg to 0.3 mg. I do, however, feel a moderately intense burning pain in my right chest, so it's probably a good idea to get some medication IV until I know I can tolerate oral.

But this entire time, almost in and out of consciousness, I am also thinking, *Where's Paul? I need to see Paul. Where is he? Why isn't he back here yet?* It must be a very strong psychological need to see family as soon as possible, coming out of surgery, and be able to say "Hey, it's over! I made it through!" After some time but what seems like forever, they usher him back in. He brings me a vase of flowers and a box of chocolates. It's funny because this is a same-day operation and I am actually going to leave the hospital around 3:00 p.m., just eight hours after arrival. But these gifts are not really for the hospital stay; it's for the fact that it is our anniversary. I thank him and smile. Why, it's dark chocolate sea salt caramels, my favorite. I had dropped major hints to him that our hospital gift shop carries these Abdullah confections as well as a nice selection of fresh flowers.

Next, I am so incredibly thirsty. My mouth feels like cotton. I devour a cup of ice chips, then another, then ask for soda—a Diet Coke sounds terrific. They bring me Diet Shasta; fine, anything at this point. An eight-ounce can, followed by another. I'm now fully awake, feeling pretty good actually. Minimal pain. Absolutely no nausea. Dr. Iannazzo was right! These guys are brilliant. I get up to get dressed. My legs feel a little wobbly but nothing like after I had an epidural.

Flashback: Despite my labor and delivery nurse telling me, "Don't get up, please don't get up. Use your call button," right after she leaves the room, I need to get up and use the bathroom. I can feel my legs. I can move them around in the bed. It's fine, right? I get up out of bed and take a step, and *womp*, down I go, land on the floor. My legs are like wet noodles. Then I lose control of my bladder, and I can't get up. I'm lying in a puddle of my own urine, completely humiliated and helpless. I have to call for the nurse, and she storms back into the room with the most angry look on her face.

Fast-forward: Well, not nearly as bad, not even close, this time. I can get dressed with minimal assistance. The RN and nursing assistant keep me company; they ask questions, make small talk, and want to see pictures of my kids. The shift change is at 3:00 p.m.; the next RN has a pretty easy job, simply presenting me with my discharge papers and instructions. I think, *If they are sending me home that quickly, it must have gone well. It's all good.*

I am wheeled down to the front lobby by transport. Paul has to go back to my ramp and get the car. We didn't use the valet; we used my high-priced contract parking instead. As I am sitting there for about twenty minutes in sweatpants and a fleece jacket with the flowers in my lap, I see familiar faces passing me by—several doctors and one of my patients that I know well who also works here. They are definitely recognizing me, but I simply smile weakly and say nothing. I'm just so happy it is over and relieved to be going home.

Later, I would pause and reflect on how the memories surrounding my time in the OR were so crisp, so distinct, filled with detail—and this is despite general anesthesia, benzodiazepines, opioid pain medication. I have got to believe it's the sheer stress of having surgery, the high level of adrenaline, and so on. Epinephrine has been shown to augment laying down of memories. But as a health-care provider myself, it reminds me to always think of the patient first even while they are under sedation or general anesthesia. It would be best to consider them "awake," still truly a part of the operation or procedure. Because clearly, I *heard* the comments coming from the team in the PACU even before I was fully conscious and able to interact with them. Another interesting observation that I would carry with me going forward.

After getting into the car and pulling away from the valet zone, I start to realize that I am actually feeling quite hungry, which makes sense—having nothing to eat since yesterday evening. I mention this to Paul. Since our kids are with our after-school nanny until 6:00 pm., he suggests stopping by one of our favorite restaurants in the neighborhood on the way home, Chianti Grill. I'm feeling up for it; the hunger pangs are definitely much stronger and more bothersome than the very minimal post-op pain I'm experiencing. We park the car and are walking across the parking lot when who do I see but my mom strolling across the same parking lot with a Barnes & Noble shopping bag in her hand!

Mom had driven down from our home town of Milaca the night before and was going to stay with me for the next few days in case I needed any help or just moral support and company. The funny thing is, I did not tell her to meet at Chianti Grill, and I hadn't even gotten the chance yet to call or text her any updates—but here we are, the three of us meeting up in the parking lot as if nothing ever happened, or as if it were a lunch date planned weeks ago! She glances over our way, and then I see her smile and laugh. She picks up her pace to come over and give me a big hug. She's truly amazed to see me standing here and starts marveling at how well everything went and how quickly I was discharged to home. We go inside the restaurant and are seated at a booth; Mom and Paul order wine to celebrate, but I stick with iced tea, following Dr. Tuttle's post-op instructions to the letter.

For our early dinner, I order my Chianti favorite, Zuppa di Pesce—a lovely seafood stew in a tomato-based broth with plenty of garlic, basil, limoncello, and a wonderful grilled flatbread on the side. After the server sets the very generous-sized bowl in front of me, I stare at the steaming broth with shrimp, scallops, and salmon floating inside it, along with tender-crisp bright green asparagus and earthy portobello mushrooms. I inhale deeply, savoring the aroma. It is pure bliss. I don't think any food tasted better to me in my entire life than those first few bites.

Going forward, whenever we order food from Chianti Grill—which is quite often, we are definitely regulars—glancing over the menu, I will always read the description of Zuppa di Pesce, listed as one of their signature dishes, and smile. *First meal after surgery.* It's the start of several miniature milestones—first meal, first day back at work, first run, first golf outing, first holiday, the list goes on. I also seem to have a new appreciation for the simple pleasures in life, such as an ice-cold Diet Coke, tasting a delectable bowl of seafood after not eating for over eighteen hours, or getting to go home and sleep in your own bed on post-op day zero.

As the saying goes, sometimes it's the little things. I'm truly grateful for all this, and so much more.

Chapter 13

RECOVERY TIME

Physician, heal yourself.
—Luke 4:23

I have been given two weeks off work to recover from surgery. Now, I haven't had more than seven consecutive days off since my maternity leave with Lydia nine years ago. To me, this seems luxurious. A spa retreat, only at home. Initially, I felt pretty good, other than some fatigue. I took lots of power naps during the first week, or should I say cat naps. My orange tabby cat, Harvey, lies on my lap most of the time, purring, so happy that I am at the house all day long. Pain is really quite minimal. Dr. Tuttle was right, predicting I would bounce back fairly quickly.

My mom stays with me the first four days; she is amazing, doing the dishes, running loads of laundry, helping with the kid's routines. We also get to talk, visit over coffee, and even do a little shopping. After all, I obviously need new lingerie. I find the perfect brassiere for me now is actually an athletic bra with removable pads. They are removable in the sense that they are basically two round, disc-shaped foam pads tucked inside a soft pocket sewn inside each cup. I can take them both out or place two or more in the right pocket or whatever else is needed. These athletic bras are available at every department store, not just Mastectomies R Us. Inexpensive, too. I grew up in a very modest-income household, every penny squeezed, and to this day, I am somewhat of a bargain shopper. No way am I paying over $100 for some specialized post-surgery bra. And I also marvel at how much my perspective has changed. I used to resent being an A cup; now, I love it because it is so easy to create symmetry! Definitely don't need a plastic surgeon for that!

My church friends bring over some meals—a Crock-Pot of beef stew, a chicken-and-rice casserole, a pan of enchiladas, all kinds of baked goodies, from banana bread to bars to homemade chocolate chip cookies. I am almost feeling guilty about all this. I'm not supposed to lift anything greater than ten pounds, but I could probably prepare a meal without too much difficulty. Mom reminds me that I have baked lasagna and brought it to a new mom at church and I took a pot roast to a family who lost their dad to lymphoma. It's time for me to accept something in return, she says. Well, okay.

As far as pain management, I have new perspectives on that too. I was sent home with that oxycodone. There are, unfortunately, so many patients who go to great lengths to obtain this type of medication. I stare at the bottle, and instead of pain relief, I am thinking, *Urinary retention, ileus, brain fog—I don't want to take any of it*. I recall taking one Vicodin after having wisdom teeth extraction in my twenties, and it made me sleep the entire day. So I start with scheduled extra-strength Tylenol, which I haven't taken in years. I do better with NSAIDs, but I was told to avoid due to bleeding risk. I am pleasantly surprised that it works great. Now, let me tell you, most patients I see with chronic pain always state that Tylenol doesn't work. They get GI upset from NSAIDs and have an allergic reaction to gabapentin and tramadol. I might sound cynical here, but I start to think, *They may be just be deluding themselves*.

But at night, things get just a little shaky. There is a saying in medicine residency: "Everything gets worse at night." It is, like most clichés, amazingly true. Whether it's pain, fever, delirium, hypotension, you name it—whatever the patient is experiencing, it is worse at 2:00 a.m. That is why the cross-cover pager goes off constantly—to alert the doctor who is least familiar with the patient's care that the crap is hitting the proverbial fan. Cross-cover was never for the faint of heart; I am glad that in recent years, it has largely been replaced by night float. At least the same night-float resident is working night shifts, usually at least one week, often two or more in a row. They get to know the patients, as opposed to a rotating call schedule. Terrible for circadian rhythm but better for patient care. At least, that is what we in academic medicine think, and we have gone to great lengths to implement in our training programs. And we have to comply with those duty-hour restrictions after all.

But here in our master bedroom suite, I don't have the nurse call button or the night float to help me out. I wake up at 2:00 a.m. on the second night with a searing pain in my right chest. It's like a hot poker is in the right armpit. It feels so very strange. I lay awake in bed for a while, observing the symptoms. There are other odd sensations on my chest wall too. It feels like crawling, tingling, or a bag of worms moving around, or at one point, as if two fingers are dragging across the incision. I am wondering what on earth is happening. Are some of these nerves, deadened by trauma or local anesthetic, just starting to wake up? I realize, lying there, that the hot-poker-burning-type pain is actually coming from the drain site. I start to think, *Maybe I should look into this.* I get up, go into the bathroom, and turn on the lights.

I'm all bandaged up and have one of those nice, soft athletic bras over it for bedtime, so it takes me some time to get undone. I inspect the incision—looks clean, a bit of soft tissue swelling, but no ecchymoses, no drainage. I check out the drain site. A very small red rim is visible on the skin surface where it is sutured in, but again, no purulent drainage. The drain bulb itself has its usual amber-colored fluid inside, a small amount. I think, *Did I just accidentally pull on the tube while turning over in my sleep?* At least it does not appear dislodged or out of place. I wonder if I have a fever. I take my temp. No, it's 98.5.

Now, Paul is awake and comes in the bathroom to make sure everything is okay. He stares a bit at my completely exposed chest, then looks away. I know things like this are sometimes too much for him. He's not medically trained. He's a bit squeamish. I guess I can't blame him for that.

But now it's almost 3:00 a.m. and I don't know what to do. Certainly, this is no reason to contact the on-call surgery resident;

everything based on my assessment seems to be in working order. I'm back in cross-cover mode. *This can wait until morning until the primary team takes over.* I take out that bottle of oxycodone and think, *Well, maybe this is the time for it.* Paul agrees with me; he doesn't like the look of distress on my face.

I swallow one 5 mg tablet with a little bit of water. It doesn't take long, and I feel the pain evaporating, but also, it totally knocks me out. I fall into a deep, dreamless sleep until 8:30 a.m. the next morning. My eyelids feel heavy, so very heavy. It takes me a long time to wake up and shake off the fog. How can people get addicted to this stuff? In the light of dawn, though, as opposed to at night, it's always better. The sun is shining, and the birds are chirping. It's a beautiful spring morning. I go back to the Tylenol, and luckily, I never needed the oxycodone again.

In the coming days, I feel my energy level coming back; I skip the napping. After five days, pain is practically gone other than these itchy, prickly, slightly sharp sensations from time to time, but they are fleeting. I stop all the meds. The warm spring weather allows me to take long walks; I gradually increase until I am walking my entire three-mile running route around Lake Como and back. Although it's just not the same as running, I find it very therapeutic and somewhat more interesting because I notice so many more things around me. The flowering crab tree, the lilac in bloom, the grape hyacinth pushing through the dirt. The tulips and daffodils. Ducks and geese. The warble of a meadowlark. I pass a fallen tree jutting out from the water and count not one, not two, but five turtles sunning themselves on that log.

I also hear, sadly, the ping of a golf club hitting a tee shot walking by the Como golf course. This is absolutely perfect weather for playing golf; sunny, sixty degrees, you won't overheat. You can walk and carry your clubs for exercise without breaking a sweat. I miss this almost as much as I miss running. Golf is also really the only "date night" that Paul and I enjoy. Sure, we play, but we also talk and catch up on things in between each hole or while waiting on the tee box for the next group at a par 3. I'm really a hack, not that great of a player, but I can get myself around any course; I have good golf etiquette, which goes a long way. I usually par a couple of holes and have maybe one great drive that keeps me coming back for more. That's how golf is; it's an impossible game to master unless you devote tons of time to it, but once you start, you sort of can't stop.

Oh well, I thought, *at least it's early. There is a possibility that I will be back at it for the second half of the season.* The Ryder Cup is also going to be hosted here at Hazeltine in September; that would be a fabulous outing if we can get tickets. I am finding that it's good to have goals, to have things to look forward to. After one week, I even start looking forward to going back to work. *Well*, I think, *at least I must be in the right profession if I am feeling this way.*

But then I also realize that I am still waiting on some important test results, including the pathology report and that Oncotype assay; I need to see Dr. Tuttle back next Thursday for a post-op check, then later Dr. Blaes. I remind myself to take this one day at a time, one foot in front of the other. I'm just grateful for the smooth recovery thus far.

Chapter 14

A New Song Gets
Stuck in My Head

And someone saved my life tonight, sugar bear.
—Elton John

S unday evening, May 1, it's a little after 8:00 p.m. Kids are
already in pajamas, winding down; it's the start of the
school week tomorrow. I have been in and out of the EMR
all weekend because I'm on call for the clinic and had to perform
a few minor tasks. I also realize I forgot to co-sign my resident's
notes right before I went on leave, and I just got a friendly reminder
from our billing and coding people to do that. I finish a few dot-
phrase attestations while I am in still logged in.

I look at the calendar beside my desk. Dr. Tuttle had said the
pathology should be back by Friday or Monday; I've been growing
more anxious by the day. Since I have access to my own chart, and
here I am, gee-whiz, logged into the EMR anyway, I think, *Do I
dare look? Should I view this alone or wait for someone from his office
to call me?* After thinking it through, I just can't resist; I decide, of
course, on the former. I type my own name into the patient search
button, open my chart, go to the Results tab, and I see "Surgical
Pathology Exam: Final Result." Oh my, it's back.

I let out a long, slow breath. I wasn't really worried about
the surgical margins, given the small size of the tumor, but
you just never know—sometimes there can be nipple or skin

involvement, which is not obvious. The presence or absence of any lymph node metastasis also affects not only treatment (I'm hoping I won't need axillary radiation) but long-term prognosis. The nodes appeared benign on the MRI imaging, but still, Dr. Tuttle quoted a 15 percent chance that there would be lymph node involvement. And in the weeks leading up to surgery, I had felt a twinge of pain in my right armpit. At first, I thought it was because I had swung a golf club for the first time in six months; then I began to fear: *Oh no, it's those lymph nodes reacting to some tumor cells showing up.*

I click on the report, which opens up on the screen, and start to scroll through it, barely able to breathe.

Final diagnosis:
B: Right breast, simple mastectomy:
- Invasive lobular carcinoma, Nottingham grade 2, size 12 mm, at 1:00
- Invasive ductal carcinoma, Nottingham grade 2, size 7 mm, at 12:30
- Ductal carcinoma in situ (DCIS), nuclear grade 2, solid type with lobular involvement
- DCIS is admixed with and adjacent to invasive ductal carcinoma and comprises approximately 15 percent of that tumor.
- Lobular carcinoma in situ (LCIS), classical type
- LCIS is admixed with invasive lobular carcinoma and is adjacent to invasive lobular and invasive ductal carcinoma.

So that is how these two tumors got started, possibly transforming from DCIS/LCIS to invasive. I pause and wonder, *How long have they been there? When did that invasive transformation actually occur?*

"You almost had your hooks in me, didn't you, dear?"

Final diagnosis, B: continued
- No lymphovascular invasion identified
- Benign nipple and skin
- Margins are uninvolved by invasive carcinoma and DCIS.
- The non-neoplastic breast shows fibrocystic change.

A sigh of relief. "Sweet freedom whispered in my ear."

Then on to the nodes. Dr. Tuttle had sent three in total, not just one, fitting just perfectly with that three-part refrain.

C: Lymph node, right axillary, sentinel #1, excision:
- One benign lymph node (0/1)

"Someone saved . . ."

D: Lymph node, right axillary, sentinel #2, excision:
- One benign lymph node (0/1)

"Someone saved . . ."

E: Lymph node, right axillary, sentinel #3, excision:
- One benign lymph node (0/1)

"Someone saved my life tonight."

Lymph Nodes Synoptic Summary
Total Number of Lymph Nodes Examined: 3
Micro/Macro Metastases: Not identified
Number of Lymph Nodes with Isolated Tumor Cells: None
Sentinel Lymph Nodes Examined: 3
Method of Evaluation: H&E, multiple levels

I am filled with intense joy. My eyes well up with tears. From what I know right now, at this moment in time, it's gone. I am cancer-free, and I bask in that moment of jubilation. "Fly away, high away, bye, bye . . ."

I let out a shout from the basement, and my poor family wonders what on earth is going on, not having told them what I was up to down below. I run up the stairs and drag them all back down to the computer and read off these results to them. Whether they fully understand the technical terms or not, they can see my obvious elation; we all cheer and laugh and hug. Then I go back up the stairs to the piano and dig out the Elton John Anthology, and I say to Paul, "Maestro, play this tune." I know I am acting crazy, but I just don't care.

And besides, that Bernie Taupin could really write a song.

Chapter 15

THE POST-OP APPOINTMENT

A surgeon reaches maturity only when he stops taking himself too seriously; some will never reach this phase.

I 've been on cloud nine since reviewing the pathology report, but I honestly can't wait to see Dr. Tuttle on Thursday for one major reason: getting that blasted drain out. I've been online looking at various sources of information; some patients describe having a drain in place for two, three weeks or more. I'm praying, "Please God, no." It's such a pain. Literally (as in that night I described earlier) as well as figuratively. How do you shower with this thing in? I had to think about it for a while; I made a lanyard with a clean white shoelace, one that Sam pulled out of his basketball shoes to replace with a different color. I place it around my neck and hang the bulb from it to prevent gravity from dragging it down. Then I enter the shower. Also, the drain is definitely limiting my wardrobe options. I have to wear tops with ruffles or a peplum, or I have to layer on a cardigan to hide the drain.

I've been checking the drain output, and it has been really scant, less than 10 cc per twenty-four hours for several days now. I have a thought cross my mind: *I could easily pull this drain myself.* I still have a few surgical instruments and supplies at home, including a needle driver, 4-0 Vicryl, sterile scissors, a suture removal kit. Back in the day, I used to practice on pillows for suturing up lacerations on patients in the ER. I still can tie a one-handed surgical square knot, which, believe it or not, really comes in handy for so many other tasks, from wrapping Christmas presents to sewing a hole in my kids' favorite stuffed animal. And I can always resort to an instrument tie if the thread gets too short.

But no, I am perfectly aware. This drain is my surgeon's territory, and I would never disrespect him that way. I patiently put up with this awkward appendage dangling from my chest wall to around my waist on the right side. Also, Lydia—a.k.a., home visiting nurse—is fascinated with this drain. She checks it every day, sometimes two to three times a day, and asks me if it is normal that the fluid appears blood tinged or amber. I can't help but think about how these experiences are shaping them for some possible future events or maybe even career paths, for better or worse. But I also don't believe trying to hide things from our children is helpful either. They are extremely perceptive and have very big ears, no sense in even trying.

The morning of the appointment, Sam and Lydia are having breakfast at the kitchen table. I say, "Great news, kids! I will probably get this drain out today! Hooray!"

Sam asks, "But will it hurt?"

I say, "Probably not, and if it does, it's only for a second, like when you have to tear a bandage off really fast. It hurts, but then it's all done."

He looks at me with a brooding, rather teenage expression and just says, "Worse." I laugh. I am trying not to think about it that way, but I did anticipate it could possibly be painful. I take another two extra-strength Tylenol an hour before the appointment, just in case.

I drive to work (I mean clinic), my same familiar route, and check in at 8:11 a.m. for the 8:30 a.m. visit. I wait for a few minutes outside clinic 2B, reviewing PowerPoint slides on my tablet for an upcoming talk, and then get called back to check vital signs and be placed in a room. The assistant asks me to undress, change into a gown from the waist up, and have a seat on the exam table. I think, *So soon?* I like greeting people in my street clothes first. I never make my own patients change into a gown before talking with them for the same reason; some dignity is a good thing. But then I realize, having surgery is just, well, different. What is the point of modesty after being completely naked in the OR and under general anesthesia to boot?

There's a knock, and in walks Dr. Todd Tuttle with a medical student. I sit up and shake his hand, then shake the hand of the student. I am grinning from ear to ear. "You look great!" he says. "I *feel* great!" I respond. Now, I barely remember seeing him post-op. With some anesthesia on board, I didn't even recall what he had said to me, but later, he obviously sent me home same day, so I knew the procedure must have gone well in his mind. "How are you doing?" he asks. "Any pain?"

I tell him, "No, I only took two oxycodone out of that thirty-tablet supply, and I've been doing fine with extra-strength Tylenol ever since."

"So," he says, "you are not going the way of our Purple Prince."

This is actually a very sad side note. The amazing musical talent Prince was found dead at his home on April 21, 2016, at the age of fifty-seven. The entire state of Minnesota was in mourning. Our Guthrie Theater, the Stone Arch bridge, the IDS building—they all lit up in purple at night. As a child of the '80s, I could recall the album *Purple Rain* as one of my very first music purchases, shortly after Duran Duran and the Go-Go's. That day, hearing the news, I remember thinking, *Prince is dead. I have cancer. The world is simply coming to an end.* Shortly after, reports started surfacing that he might have overdosed on Percocet. Again, what a terrible loss yet another reason I was extremely wary of taking any narcotics.

So I tell him, "No, I don't need any more oxycodone, thank you!" I also share the story that I was actually on call for the PCC the week of surgery and didn't realize it—another reason to minimize the opioids. Although I had completely cleared my clinic patients and all my teaching duties, I had forgotten to check the night call schedule. The first evening I am home, I get a page from the Fairview Home Care nurses, and I pull up our online scheduling program. Sure enough, I'm taking call for the next four days. Now, be aware, our home call for clinic is really benign; we have a nurse advice line that screens out 80 percent of the calls, so if they do have to page us, it's something very simple, such as needing a verbal order for home care or sending a prescription to a pharmacy. It's taking call for hospital admissions that is brutal. Anyway, I had decided it was easier to just take the call than to try to find back up that late in the game.

Dr. Tuttle laughs and shares a similar story. "Maybe this is too much information," he begins, "but I had the same thing happen post vasectomy. I had a bunch of patients that I couldn't reschedule, and so I had to sit in a chair, ice pack in place, and simply talk with them. I couldn't get up and perform any examination, but somehow, I got through the day anyway." I smile and reply, "Patient seen and examined by me," which is our billing and coding way of saying, "At least I laid eyes on the patient. Now count that toward the documentation." In the days of gallows humor, we used to say, "PLGFD," which is "Patient looks good from door," sometimes the only examination performed on rounds that day in the interest of time. If this sounds too crass, remember, by a certain point, most physicians actually can tell how sick a patient is just by looking at them. It's not altogether unusual to do it this way from time to time.

The discussion then turns toward the drain. "What's been going on with the drain?" he asks. I show him the bulb; there is maybe 5 cc in it, at most, and I tell him this has been the only output since I showered at noon yesterday. "Oh, that's good. Maybe we only need to leave it in another week or two." I had been fiddling with it when I abruptly stop and look up.

He starts laughing, his green eyes twinkling. "I'm kidding!" I must have appeared totally crestfallen. "You should have seen the look on your face!" he says. Now, we are both laughing; I am glad we can joke around at this point. I had attempted humor with him on the morning of surgery, but I was way too nervous to pull it off. The med student is just standing in the corner, taking this all in.

So now it's on to the physical exam. I think the incision looks great, myself, but it would have to be spewing pus for me to know anything was going on. I just don't see these early post-op incisions or follow wound healing or anything even close in my own practice. There's an old doctor joke that goes, "How do you hide a hundred dollar bill from an internist? Place it under a dressing." Precisely.

And the exam, for me, is the slightly awkward part, so I am talking all the while to fill a void; I tell him I wanted to thank him in particular for his level-headed, even-tempered, evidence-based approach to my situation despite my emotional ups and downs (such as the panic text I sent him requesting a bilateral mastectomy). He pauses, his facial expression changes to a kind and sympathetic look, and he says, "*I don't think you were being unreasonable at all.*" I tell him my mind assumed the worst at every turn. "That's your physician brain working against you. You know too much." It is just then that I realize, by golly, he's already taken the drain out, and I didn't even notice. Not a twinge of pain! Strong work.

I sit back up and cover up with the gown. "I do need to run a few things by you, activity-wise." I tell him, "I'm getting on a plane to Baltimore, and you can read horror stories on the internet—urban legend, probably, of mastectomy incisions opening up and draining due to the pressure changes."

"When are you going to Baltimore?"

"Ten days from now," I say.

"That should be fine. How long are you there?"

"Three days."

He smiles again. Then I remember, when I was checking out his credentials, I saw he went to medical school at Johns Hopkins—that is exactly where I will be presenting at a national meeting come May 16. "Your old stomping grounds!" I say. "Can you recommend any restaurants?"

He smiles, another twinkle in his eye, and says, "Not restaurants but certainly bars. I did a lot of damage in Baltimore." He recommends that I check out Fell's Point, especially the oldest drinking establishment in America, now known as the Horse You Came in On Saloon. He describes the local pub scene there back in the day, listening to cover bands of Van Morrison and other live music, with fellow medical students and surgery residents. I tell him, "That sounds great. I'll be sure to stop by."

Next, I just have to bring up exercise. I tell him, "I've been walking three miles a day, and while it's been great, I sure do miss running."

He is looking at the computer and turns to me to ask, "When was your surgery date again?"

I tell him, "April 26, nine days ago."

"Oh yes, of course. I mean, *no*. You can definitely not run yet, not for a couple more weeks. You can walk at a brisk pace to start."

I say, "Well, that's good enough." Inwardly: *I think the track or the treadmill would be okay, even now, much less impact than running outside.*

He goes on to say, "You saw the path report, I presume, which was good news!" Yes, I tell him, I was elated to see that report. I neglected to mention that my new nickname for him is Sugar Bear; he might find that a bit odd. Although, honestly, he seems like a hip-enough guy to get the obscure Elton John musical reference.

He tells me the Oncotype assay—that specialized test which essentially dictates chemo or no chemo—is still pending and might be for another week or so. I mention I have a follow-up appointment with Dr. Blaes, and I will keep looking for any new results in Epic. "Susan will call you too," he says to reassure me. "Susan pretty much runs the show around here." (Ah, she's his version of my Tony.)

It's about time to wrap up the appointment. I ask, "Do I need to see you back?"

He explains "Not unless there is a problem. You always know how to get a hold of me."

I shake his hand and shake hands again with the medical student. I'm still smiling and just so pleased with everything, and I *especially* enjoy getting dressed again without working around that darn drain. I am gathering up my belongings when I hear another knock, and Susan enters the room.

"It's great to see you! I'm glad to hear you are doing so well!" She's smiling at me; she has wavy dark-brown hair and warm and friendly brown eyes. She is dressed in fun, brightly patterned pink scrubs and a black fleece warm-up jacket that sports the pink ribbon for breast cancer awareness. Her dark-purple horn-rimmed glasses have sparkly pink glitter inserts at each temple. For a second, I think, *It must be professionally rewarding to practice in such a specialized, focused area that you can devote almost all your time and energy to one cause, one disease, even to the point of dressing the part.* I then realize that I am wearing a pale-pink sweater today over dark jeans, and the thought hadn't even occurred to me about the new meaning of that color.

"Thank you, Susan, for all your help, your phone calls and updates, and everything," I say. Then I exit the 2B clinic, passing Dr. Tuttle and his student working in the collaboration zone, and go upstairs to my 4B clinic to say hello.

Later on, I am back in my office. I thought to myself, *I'm so very grateful for the amazing care I just received.* What a great team. But honestly, it seems odd that I won't need to see surgery again; now, all my follow-up will be transferred over to oncology. The usual, I know, but still, it feels a bit abrupt.

I decide to open my desk drawer. In it, I have yet another collection of blank cards, including some humorous, some holiday-themed, some thank-you notes and such, in case I forget that it's National Nurses Day or Administrative Assistant Day or just feel the need to send someone a note. I've even sent some to the physicians who volunteer to teach in my course; I have found that a handwritten note inside an artistic card goes a long way in this age of impersonal e-mail.

I heard later from Dr. Berryman that Dr. Marsh very much appreciated that card from me earlier this month. And I've gotten cards, books, other gifts from my patients over the years; just recently, I was given a painting from a woman, a longtime patient of mine whom I sent to cath lab. I recognized she was having an MI in my clinic based on some very vague symptoms and some subtle EKG changes. The stat troponin confirmed what I feared. Now, every time I see her, she hugs me and thanks me for saving her life. She doesn't even remember the cardiologist who performed the angiogram and the stent, who *technically was* the person who saved her life; it's me and my nurse, Tony, that she admires for hitting the appropriate panic buttons, stat paging cardiology, activating the cath lab, and even wheeling her over ourselves to the second-floor interventional area. She's a painter and brought me a watercolor of an underwater scene, bright-yellow tropical fish in a background of deep blues and dark-green seaweed. That painting holds tons of meaning for me. Upon presenting it to me, I thank her; and knowing she's also one of those beloved aging hippie types, I tell her, "How did you know

I was a Pisces?" (Which I am, by the way.) She smiles: "Really! I am a Gemini!"

So I decide, I sure can't paint a watercolor, but a thank-you note is the least I can do. I find a blank card that begins with a child's quote; it's an out-of-the-mouths-of-babes sort of theme. On the front, it says in a child's handwriting, "Life is like a roller coaster. It goes up and down, it makes you scream, and it costs a lot to ride." Perfect. I address the outside envelope: "Dr. Todd Tuttle and Susan Pappas-Varco." Inside I write:

> Thank you both for helping me up the first "big hill" on this roller coaster ride.
>
> With sincere gratitude,
> Heather Thompson Buum

Chapter 16

THE MENTOR (PART II)

The only people with whom you should try to "get
even" are those who have helped you.
—John Southard

The very next morning (I cannot make this stuff up), a new
twist and turn develops on this ride. I did eventually
send that card to Dr. Tuttle and his nurse Susan, but the
next day, I was also sending him yet another text message for an
entirely different reason.

I went for my morning walk around Lake Como, and at
around 9:30 a.m., I am just getting back to the house when I see an
unfamiliar number on both my pager and my mobile phone. I've
been returning so many different types of calls over the past few
weeks that I decide I had better figure out who this is. I dial the
number, and it's actually Charles Moldow.

"Go and look me up in Epic. I give you permission to review
my path report." Now, I knew Charlie was having surgery the
same week as me; he had been joking all along about this, about
how we should be meeting up in the recovery room and something
about the fact that, anatomically, his surgery is happening at the
opposite end of the human body. I put that together with the fact
that he will need sitz baths and might be unable to sit down, and
I assume he's having hemorrhoid surgery. I don't ask about the
details; he promises not to show me his scar.

But today, he's obviously worried about something. He's rambling a bit as I finally get the EMR loaded on my tablet and get his name entered into the search bar and click on the path report.

"What? Merkel cell carcinoma?" I say into the phone.

"What the heck? I can barely remember what that is. But holy crap, this is not what I would have expected!" he says. "You are sounding just like Greg Vercellotti." (An oncology colleague we both know quite well.)

In a split second, while he's going on about needing a PET CT, I type into Google, and I find out this is a rare and pretty aggressive form of skin cancer, sort of like melanoma. "How can I get skin cancer where the sun doesn't shine?" he asks. That is a very good point. I see in Google Scholar a recent trial of a monoclonal antibody therapy in *The New England Journal of Medicine,* and the survival curves are measured in months, not years . . . holy crap. In a matter of about thirty seconds, I am now more concerned about his health than my own. "What is in the water in our building?" he says. "We are all just riddled with cancer." Always trying to maintain that sense of humor. He then says, "I need to see your new favorite physician ASAP."

Who is he talking about? Dr. Tuttle? "You got it." Then I remember, well yes, he has expertise in the surgical management of melanoma, so this would be his territory for Merkel cell as well. How ironic!

But now Charlie is rambling again. "Here it is, a Friday. Of course, I can't get a hold of anyone. Tuttle is probably out of town."

I say, "No, he is not. I just saw him yesterday. He pulled my drain." Charlie responds, "Well, if you needed a drain for *that,* I'm going to need a chute." I realize that I still have Dr. Tuttle's number on my mobile phone; I ask Charlie if he would like to have it.

"Well, sure, I will write it down. I'll try not to bother him, though, unless necessary."

I mention, "I was going to work for a little while today, anyway." I ask him if he needs me to do anything while I am there. I happen to know that his usual primary MD, Dr. Jim Langland, is out of town this week, in Washington, DC, at an academic meeting. "If you need me to sign any orders or work you in for a pre-op, let me know." He says he'll call me or e-mail any updates. Before I hang up, I tell him, "Love and prayers," and he sincerely thanks me.

So I contemplate what to do. I remember exactly how I felt when I couldn't get through the call center to get that first appointment scheduled. I remember the first few days of fear, the uncertainty; I have cancer, but what does it mean? Surgery—what type? When? What about chemo? Radiation? So many questions with no answers yet. I am definitely in a much better place now, and here Charlie is right back at square one. Could I be of any assistance?

I decide to send another text to Dr. Todd Tuttle: "It's Heather again. I'm doing great. Thanks for everything. Now I wonder if you can see my mentor, Charlie Moldow, on short notice."

I then quickly shower, get dressed, and grab a protein shake to take along; and I'm out the door. As I was driving, I thought, *I didn't get a reply to that text, but Friday mornings, Dr. Tuttle is usually in clinic.* I was headed there anyway to check in with my nurse, Tony, before M&M conference at noon. Am I pestering him if I stop by? I didn't want to impose, but I thought, *After all Charlie has done for me, it seems like the least I could do. Just something, anything.*

So I wander through the clinic 2B area once again. But then I stop and think, *This is a bad idea. I'll be interrupting his clinic for no real good reason.* So instead, I make a right-hand turn to exit through the adjacent collaboration zone, and I run right into Dr. Anne Blaes.

"Hi there! How are you!" she says. She seems genuinely happy to see me.

I say, "Really good. Recovery has been going well." She's standing next to me, wearing a dark-navy pantsuit and heels, this time with her hair pulled back in a ponytail. She's so amazingly tall; I feel like a midget next to an Amazon woman.

But I have a big smile on my face again just talking to her about it; I feel as though a huge burden has been lifted, and when people ask me how I am doing, I can honestly say, "Great." Feels like a new lease on life. We both acknowledge how encouraging the path report was. We chat about how the Oncotype assay is still pending. I tell her, "I think we're on a run here of good reports coming back, and I can only assume we're on a roll." She laughs and seems to appreciate the positive attitude. She says she'll get in touch with me once those results return.

So I thank her and tell her, "I'll be seeing you soon." I am thinking, *I'll go through the back hallway and up two flights of stairs to my own clinic,* when I walk right by Dr. Todd Tuttle and the very same medical student.

"Hey there! Hello! Good to see you again!" he says.

I stop and say, "Thanks! I just ran into Anne too!" Then I decide, to heck with it: "Can I talk to you for a minute? It's not about me." We walk into an empty exam room. He sits where the patient would sit, and I sit where the physician would sit. The irony of that is not lost on me.

"Is this about Charlie?" he says. He must have gotten that text after all. "Rob also called me." He's the colorectal surgeon who performed the biopsy.

I say, "Yes, but I just have to tell you about this, how ironic it is."

I explain to him how Charlie has been a mentor to me for many years. I tell him about the sage advice, assistance with grants and manuscript review, the moral support, especially trying to teach and uphold primary care at a subspecialty-driven university. I tell him, "The ironic part is that he covered me last week for both resident clinic and student teaching to be able to have surgery, the operation you performed. Now he's asking *me* how to get in touch with *you,* and *I* will likely need to cover *him* for this upcoming surgery."

"Oh, wow," he says. I think he must agree; that's a pretty crazy coincidence.

I say, "I hope you don't mind, but I did give him your cell phone number, just in case, since I still had it. I can tell he's really nervous, and sometimes every little thing helps." I even used Charlie's term—that he was looking for my new favorite physician, Dr. Todd Tuttle. With that, just the hint of a smile plays out on his lips. Later I would think, *You know, even the chief of surgical oncology appreciates a little sincere flattery now and then.*

So I thank him for letting me barge in on him. I tell him that I was just trying to help, to repay Charlie for what he's done for me over the years. "Do you think I should call him?" he asks.

I say, "Sure, or maybe your nurse could get in touch with him."

"How old is he?" he asks.

I say, "He just retired. I think seventy-four." I can tell by his expression that he's mulling this over, thinking about fitness for surgery. I explain to him, "He's extremely active, goes to the gym, has gone skiing last month, and walks the dog for exercise. He does have an aortic valve, that's all I know for certain about his health history." So maybe this additional information is a bit helpful to him after all.

We both stand up, getting ready to leave, so I thank Dr. Tuttle again and say, "Isn't it fun taking care of physicians?"

He laughs and says, "No worries, I do this all the time."

I leave the building and walk back to Phillips-Wangensteen, where morbidity and mortality conference will be held at noon. As I am walking, I call Charlie back, telling him I spoke to Dr. Tuttle in person on his behalf.

He says, "Great! That is wonderful! Thanks for doing that. I so appreciate it. As long as I have you and Vercellotti in my court, things will happen." And then he says he now already has the PET CT scheduled for Monday and an appointment with Dr. Tuttle on Thursday. Probably this had already happened before I even showed up or said anything, but oh well. The fact that Charlie was happy and feeling reassured that we were all going the extra mile, that's what is important to me.

Chapter 17

Back to Work

Back to life, back to reality, back to the here
and now, yeah.
—Soul II Soul

Days ahead of time, I have already checked my schedule for my return; I have a slightly reduced clinic workload to help ease my way back into things. I notice that the very first patient when I am back, the 1:00 p.m. appointment on a Tuesday, is a kind and pleasant gentleman that I have been seeing since I was an intern—*in 1998*. Yes, that's eighteen years of continuity of care! I also saw his wife in clinic a few times until she developed Alzheimer's and transferred to a memory clinic. He is seventy-eight but in really good shape; his only medications are for high blood pressure. We have a great working relationship. What a blessing that I get to return to one of my all-time favorite patients! In fact, I notice that my entire schedule, the first few days back, is by and large comprised of patients I have known for five, ten years or more. This is yet another reason that, despite the new clinic building and a possible health system merger, I do not want to leave the university. I'd have to start all over again with a new panel of patients, and continuity is what makes this job so rewarding.

But I have to admit, the weekend before, I'm getting a little stressed out about going back. We try to have systems of backup, coverage if you will, while a physician is out, but it only goes so far. There is still always the backlog of forms to sign and the med refills and other patient care tasks in the EMR that will wait for you if not urgent. I'm not too worried about my physical state. Pain is nearly gone, and psychologically, I am much less anxious. However, I still have a bit of insomnia again the night before.

It's because I am going through a mental checklist of things I had left undone two weeks ago that will now need to be tended to—curriculum mapping for my second-year course, last-minute tweaking on that Baltimore presentation, meeting with a colleague and a statistician who are co-authors on a paper. It's at these times when I think how much simpler things might be if I were in private practice and not academics. Seeing patients (even very complex patients, such as post-kidney transplant, pulmonary hypertension, liver cirrhosis), I'm quite comfortable with that. It's these additional areas of teaching and research and presenting at meetings and writing manuscripts and submitting grants that pull you in so many different directions, often outside of your comfort zone. Definitely, we all wear a lot of hats, which is challenging. And while you can always attempt to find coverage for patient care tasks, you can't really find coverage for the other roles.

So knowing I am going to feel behind the very moment I walk in the front door, I drive to work and make my way to my office on the sixth floor of Mayo. I am immediately accosted by my very sweet division administrator, Suzanne. "You need to meet with Dr. Brad Benson for your annual review, and you didn't fill out the mandatory paperwork, including an individualized development plan and a list of goals for the upcoming academic year."

I think:

Staying alive.

Avoiding Docetaxel and Cytoxan if at all possible.

Keeping my sanity, as well as my hair.

Getting used to my new silhouette. It still surprises even me at times.

Tolerating tamoxifen without the disabling hot flashes, brain fog, and other terrible side effects.

She then says, "I also want to remind you to complete your online conflict of interest training."

Sadly, as usual, I say, "None to report," but then I think, *Huh, what about writing a book about my experiences and publishing it?* But poor Suzanne, she's not aware of any of this (at least I think not), so I just smile and nod. "Yes, I'll get to it right away."

I'm in my office from about 9:00 a.m. to noon, catching up on e-mail, hosting a telephone conference call, completing tasks in the EMR. Then I head over to the clinic for the 1:00 p.m. start time. And as I walk through the front door of the Clinics and Surgery Center, it's now as a physician again, not as a patient.

In the front lobby, I slow my pace, almost stopping, and glance up at the winding staircase that leads to the clinic 2B entrance. Above it, I see the bold lettering: The Masonic Cancer Clinic. The Breast Center. I still have a hard time believing even now that this applies to *me*. Going forward, every time I walk through the front door of my own building (sometimes multiple times a day), I will glance up and look at those signs. It's a bittersweet reminder. I'm still grateful; I have so much to be thankful for. But life is a bit different since this diagnosis, always will be—not a bad thing necessarily, just different. And now I have to admit, for what it's worth, I'm even starting to *like* this new building, at least certain parts of it. I'm growing attached to it, I guess, both as doctor and patient.

I connect with Tony first. He says, "Welcome back! Ready to jump in and see patients this afternoon?" He gives me updates on the important things that happened while I was away. I've already shared many stories with Tony about my recent ordeal; we've laughed about the experience of waking up from general anesthesia. He's heard about the pleasantries of having a drain in place. He hands me several narcotic refill prescriptions to sign. I jokingly say, "Who wants my leftover 28 oxycodone instead?" Since Tony is also the RN for Dr. Langland and will need to know about Charlie as his patient, I fill him on that entire situation as well. We both marvel at the remarkable coincidences and start talking about that theory, six degrees of separation. Although in reality, it's boiling down to only two or three.

One of Tony's updates involves a long-term patient of mine who is also a physician. Her name is Laurie. She's very close to me in age. Unfortunately, she's been diagnosed with a rare autoimmune disease, now with multiple complications. Some of the medications she's been on are more toxic than what I am potentially facing. Also, in the middle of all this, she was found to have an incidental renal mass, a finding on a CT of the abdomen, a spot in the kidney that turned out to be malignant. Although the lesion was small and a partial nephrectomy should be curative, well, there's all the follow-up now, including imaging studies every few months, that always seems to turn up "something." For example, the tiny pulmonary nodule that is probably nothing. Or could it be metastatic renal cell carcinoma? I've been trying to help her navigate all this, and I find myself thinking, *Wow, now I know exactly where she is coming from.* The anxiety, the fear, the over-interpretation of every finding, assuming the worst. All that medical training now constantly working against you.

Tony says, "Laurie seems a bit anxious about your being gone, keeps asking, 'What is happening?' 'Are you okay?' 'When are you coming back?'" I start to think about it from her perspective; I've been her primary doc for many years, and hers is a complicated story. I would not, in her shoes, want to start all over again with another physician. It's also probably quite concerning for any patient to hear that their *doctor* might be facing some serious health issues. They are supposed to be healers, not the ones battling illness themselves! It's at that point I mention, "Next time I see her in the office, I may just share with her what's been going on." I've been contemplating doing that anyway; there may be some benefit to opening up to selected patients, putting it all out there, allowing some vulnerability and authenticity to pervade our doctor-patient relationship. This is something very new for me. I would have never thought this way before—other than I did make many connections with my female patients who were also mothers after I became a mom myself. We would commiserate about the painful stuff—colic, breastfeeding woes, sleepless nights—and share some of the mutually beneficial observations.

So now, I am contemplating a whole new experience, a potential opportunity in sharing my cancer diagnosis. I know this is very different from bonding over child rearing. I have my own thoughts, ideas, and impressions about how this may play out; but of course, it's all so new. It's definitely venturing into uncharted territory. I am hoping it can somehow work together for good.

Romans 8:28 says, "All things work together for good to those that love God." As my husband has pointed out before, it doesn't say *all things* are good—it says all things *work together* for good. Cancer isn't good. A heart attack isn't good. Divorce isn't good. Mental illness isn't good. Addiction isn't good. Slowly losing a parent to Alzheimer's isn't good. But the promise is to simply hold on and persevere until these things can work together to accomplish something even greater than what we would be without them.

Chapter 18

More Test Results

Only in medicine is a negative test result considered a
positive thing, and vice versa.

I have my follow-up appointment with Dr. Anne Blaes moved
to May 23 so that we can be sure all the necessary tests are
back prior to the visit. Leading up to that appointment,
several important results return, and I have been contemplating
the meaning of them.

First, I am obviously a phenotype, not a genotype. My panel
of genetic testing—yes, all seventeen mutations that I opt for in a
moment of sheer insanity—comes back negative. I have not even
one mutated gene out of the seventeen tested that I can blame for
having this cancer.

On the other hand, I humbly accept that information, and I'm
not too surprised. I must share something that occurred ten or more
years ago right after Sam was born. Paul and I were applying for life
insurance; we had a nurse come to our house. She checked our blood
pressure, measured our height and weight, and drew a bunch of
labs. Based on that, I got the "very super high excellent rating," and
Paul just the "high excellent rating." Not caring too much, we get
to purchase the life insurance, with a substantial benefit to Sam at
a reasonable cost. But I have to admit, having this sort of evaluation
makes you contemplate when or how you will die.

[More than ten years ago.]
ME: I think if I die from anything, it will be from breast cancer.
PAUL: Why do you think that?
ME: Well, according to my labs, my cholesterol, and BMI, I will
be struck by lightning before I will have a heart attack or
develop diabetes. And statistically speaking, it's the most
common cancer for women. I just have a feeling, that's all.

[Fast-forward ten-plus years.]
ME: Paul, I have to tell you. I found a lump in my breast, and I am
going to have a mammogram today.
PAUL: Is this just your paranoia that you are going to get breast
cancer?
ME: No. [*Pause, awkward silence.*]

Again, doctors love being right. This time, I hate being right.
Somehow, I had put it together, years ago even. But then, it's really
not that hard; it's a pretty good guess when you consider my
demographic:
White, Western female.
Early-ish menarche.
Chose to have children in her mid-thirties instead of earlier.
Breastfed the absolute bare minimum. (Three months each
until I went back to work, and that was enough of that! Isn't this
why we invented formula?)
Will enjoy a glass or two of wine with dinner.
Very dense breasts (first on exam, later confirmed on
imaging).
These are all risk factors for developing breast cancer. I most
definitely fit the phenotype, if not the genotype. What about
Oncotype?
Remember, I'm waiting on that Oncotype assay, the high-
tech testing performed on the tumor itself, to predict the risk of
recurrence and decide on chemotherapy. I get a call on my cell
phone at 12:45 p.m., my first day back at work, as I am on the
shuttle going over to the Clinics and Surgery Center. I didn't want
to pick up and take the call since the shuttle was full, so I waited
until I stepped off and walked outside to listen to the new voice

mail. "Heather, it's Susan calling. I have some very good news about your Oncotype result. Call me back at 612-676-5200."

I call her back right away. She is happy to inform me that my Oncotype score is 4. "What on earth does that mean?" I ask. I have absolutely no clue. Apparently, 0–18 is low risk, 18–32 intermediate, and anything above 32, high risk. The range is 0–100; my score is 4, *as in four*, single digits. This translates to a ten-year recurrence rate of about 5 percent if I take tamoxifen. Apparently, I have a better chance of getting hit by a bus. And very importantly, she says, "Chemotherapy is generally not recommended given this result."

I am thrilled, and I tell her, "Well, you know the saying, 'You never want to be an interesting case at a teaching hospital.' I must be the most boring case you guys have seen in a while!"

She laughs. I thank her for the update; I am very happy to hear this news, almost as elated as seeing that path report.

So tamoxifen it is. This will be a good drug for my particular case, no doubt. Then *(here we go)* I start to ponder the situation a bit more. I think about the fact that my tumors are both strongly estrogen receptor positive. Now, keep in mind, I teach a pathophysiology course in the second year of medical school; I am trained to think, to ask my students, "What is exactly the mechanism of this disease?" So I can't help it. I start to apply this to myself and consider estrogen in general and its myriad of effects, and I come up with this list.

Early twenties: We were learning how to draw blood in medical school, and we got to submit it for free cholesterol screening. I had a cholesterol panel that showed a pretty high HDL, and I was really only walking to class for exercise. Estrogen tends to raise HDL.

Mid to late twenties: Had migraines with full-blown aura, only about four or five in total, but perhaps another estrogen-mediated phenomenon. Saw wavy flashing lights out of right eye, followed by visual field defect, bandlike headache. Initially, I thought I was having a stroke. Major panic and possible 911 call averted by NSAIDs and caffeine.

Early thirties: Rosacea. I flush like mad in response to certain stimuli. Research suggests estrogen may play a role. Topical creams did nothing, but laser treatments helped immensely.

Mid-thirties fertility: Both my kids were one-hit wonders, and I mean, conceived on the first attempt. While I thought it was great at the time, I also thought, *Geez! I should be more careful!* Now in retrospect, I wonder how much estrogen effect there was to allow *that* to happen at age thirty-four and thirty-six.

So apparently, I conclude, I must have a lot of circulating estrogen. I am a veritable slave to estrogen, hence the tumor. But now, I am being told to counteract its effect via tamoxifen for the next five to ten years. I think, yes, this makes sense, but at what cost? Early menopause potentially? And if I do have this many physiologic—and/or pathologic—effects of estrogen going on, what is really going to happen when I block it? Am I going to morph into a completely different person?

Hot flashes, fatigue, joint aches; these I can probably handle. What I am worried about most are the potential CNS effects. Cognitive impairment, diminished short-term recall, visual memory deficits, brain fog, all sort of names, clinical features, syndromes if you will. But it's out there—not just on the internet blogs but in the medical literature as well. I have found over the years, taking care of patients (and I would definitely agree for myself), that the prospect of losing your mental health or your mental capacity is far worse than the idea of losing your physical health. I can handle losing one breast; I can't handle losing my brain.

Then also in medical journals and plenty of air time on those patient blogs—the sexual side effects. Everything from low libido to dryness to complete anorgasmia. I grew very concerned, thinking, *Wait, I am only forty-four years old! Is this it? The end of any fun between the sheets?* And what a kick in the teeth. First, we take away your right breast, an erogenous zone, important for sexual well-being, then we must start a medication that apparently causes atrophy of everything important below the beltline.

As an aside, end of May, I received a package in clinic. Tony, my RN, approached me regarding the contents. They are drug samples that I do still get from time to time despite our practice banning them, but this time, they are Vagifem, a vaginal estrogen-replacement tablet preloaded into applicators. A whole slew of them. Tony looks at me and laughs and says, "Are you having issues with the tamoxifen?" At first, I think, *Good thing I let him in on all this. At least we can joke about it!* But truthfully, I hadn't even started taking the drug as of yet.

I say nervously, "No! Haha! Not necessary!" Then later, I secretly come back to the clinic storage cabinet and take the entire shipment home. I start to wonder, *Did I get this sent to me because I just filled a prescription for tamoxifen? Are the pharm reps privy to this kind of information? How did they know?* Or maybe it is providence.

But once again, I find that I am getting way ahead of myself. I have not even had *the second appointment yet* with Dr. Blaes; she's the expert. I know she's followed many patients on tamoxifen over the years. She'll be able to comment on possible side effects and any monitoring that needs to occur.

Then suddenly I realize, hey, even if I do get the so-called cognitive impairment, at the very least, it will stop my analytical brain from over-interpreting things every step of the way. It's the curse of the internist; I know colleagues of mine who wake up in the middle of the night and start rethinking a patient case, going over the details, wondering if they made the correct diagnosis or missed something. Maybe a very slight case of brain fog would be welcome in certain situations.

I am once again choosing to stay positive.

Chapter 19

BALTIMORE (PART I)

"I would never want to live anywhere but Baltimore; you'll
never discover a stranger city with such extreme style. It's
as if every eccentric in the South decided to move north,
ran out of gas in Baltimore, and decided to stay."
—John Waters

B eing on the faculty at a teaching hospital, I attend at least
one or two academic meetings per year. Many months
before my cancer diagnosis, I had submitted a proposal
with a colleague to a meeting called Medbiquitous, hosted
at Johns Hopkins every spring. Of course, I had no idea at the
time what was in store for me come April, and I didn't purchase
travel insurance--why would I? As a result, I found I needed to
work hard around this travel to Baltimore when I reviewed my
calendar, scheduling appointments, contemplating surgery dates,
recovery time, even possible chemotherapy. Luckily it all seemed
to fall into place.

It's my first time at this particular national meeting, which
is all about utilizing technology to improve medical education.
I actually tend to bounce around and vary which specific
conferences I attend quite a bit. Many of my colleagues are just
the opposite; they want to be sure they are always at that "one big
meeting" to get the best experience, or sometimes it is so they can
advance up the ranks in terms of a specific organization, college, or
medical society. I have a different take on it; I would rather not be
asked to serve on some planning committee, thank you. I'm busy

enough as it is. Also, maybe I am just not hard-wired to have that inner need, the desire to ascend rapidly up a ladder of leadership or recognition or promotion or whatever you may call it.

I am sure this is also a major reason why it's taken me so long to get promoted on my non-tenure teaching track—probably causing much consternation on the part of my division director, my assigned mentor, my department chair. Yet I am one of several go-to faculty members when it comes to teaching, whether it's giving a lecture, leading a small group, developing a resident as teacher curriculum, having a student with me in clinic, directing a second-year pathophysiology course, facilitating a board review course for community physicians—the list goes on and on. The problem is, those activities—no matter how numerous or how impactful—don't get you promoted. Bottom line, it's publications and grants. And if you are a general internist, seeing a ton of patients, doing lots of teaching, never involved in clinical research (but perhaps your "research" is investigating a new curriculum in the medical school or a direct observation tool in resident continuity clinic), it can be fairly challenging to get that stuff published or funded. First of all, it's "fuzzy" science; it's not a randomized clinical trial. There are no control groups. The numbers are very small; the statistical analysis seems like a joke. You submit something; and some hot-to-trot editor on the opposite end sees that right away, pokes holes in it, returns it to you, saying you need more outcomes data. Okay, fine, but if you teach a course for six weeks every fall, just once a year, it might take you decades to accumulate the kind of outcomes data they are looking for.

So I've decided to take the slow, circuitous route; I'm fine with that. Obviously, it's a non-tenure track for a reason—I could take my entire lifetime to get from assistant to associate professor! Hooray! This allows me the freedom, at least in my opinion, to take a broad approach to my work, not narrowing my focus too soon or locking down on any one specific path. I've dabbled in many different projects, leadership positions, teaching roles; and when it comes to patient care, I'm one of very few faculty members practicing both inpatient and outpatient general medicine. I'm only forty-four, and somehow, I'm old school. I'm a throwback, still not locking in as a hospitalist or primary-care doc but both.

My mentors might say I actually *lack* focus, as a criticism, and they could be right; but I have enjoyed each and every role and feel the skill sets are very complementary to one another.

It's this same approach that has led me to this meeting in Baltimore. It's called MedBiquitous; what a crazy name. I am envisioning a bunch of tech geeks, data nerds, PhD educators and doctors from all over, getting together to share ideas. The funny thing is, I am really *not* a tech geek, but I came up with an idea last year to convert some of our standard one-hour lectures in my medical school course into online learning modules. Why? I've seen lecture hall attendance dwindling over the years; most of the students are watching online anyway, so I thought, *Hey, why not try to make a better learning experience better for them?* We could use technology not just to deliver a standard PowerPoint lecture but also to incorporate practice questions, animation, video demonstrations, and other active learning to really drive home the teaching points.

Then I found my tech geek and my right-hand man in Mark Hilliard, instructional designer in the medical school. He was so enthusiastic about my idea; right away, we jointly applied for a grant from our institution and were shot down. (See? What did I just tell you? Difficult to get funded.) Undaunted, we decided to basically take our nonexistent free time and experiment with this idea in the summer of 2015. I had ten lecturers in total as willing subjects in my experiment. (Small numbers, as mentioned previously.) They recorded their standard presentation via a narrated PowerPoint with some tweaking based on my suggestions, but then Mark and I added in more fun bells and whistles at the end. We spent the better part of our days figuring out how to add animation showing the mechanism of a hepatitis C antiviral drug, or filming a faculty member using a rubber balloon to demonstrate red blood cell membrane physiology, or creating practice questions (many types of practice questions) so that the student could test what they had just learned in real time rather than waiting for the midterm or final exam to find out if they understood it.

Because this was a novel use of our existing technology, we decided to submit our work to the MedBiquitous national meeting, and our presentation gets accepted. It's my first travel since the cancer diagnosis, and it's also the first time in a long while that I am traveling alone. Last summer, I took my husband along to an academic meeting in San Diego; that's a great location for a spouse to find things to do during the day while I'm sitting in a freezing-cold hotel conference room, discussing medical school curriculum innovation. (Actually, it was that meeting that inspired me to develop the online learning modules.) I took Mom with me to a meeting before that in Chicago; she went shopping on the Magnificent Mile while I learned about ways to improve primary-care training. This time, for obvious reasons, I was really grateful to be by myself. I was looking forward to it, a mental-health break.

There is nothing quite as liberating as flying alone. It's only your carry-on bag, your boarding pass, and your personal itinerary you have to worry about. You can use your mobile instead of printing out boarding passes. You can sit anywhere; you don't need to get a window seat for the squirmy young child or an aisle seat for the husband, who will need to get up to use the bathroom. The takeoff feels as though you are leaving all cares behind. The two-and-a-half-hour flight to Baltimore, up in the clouds, with nothing but me, my thoughts, and my laptop, felt like a gift from above. And this bird has Wi-Fi! Excellent.

Once I arrive, I have a few hours to kill before Mark checks into the same hotel. We'll review our slides again in the hotel lobby; we did prepare back home for this, of course, but much less than I normally would for a national presentation. I've only been back to work four days; and the two weeks off after surgery, well, turns out I really did need some time to recover. I jokingly told Mark, "With everything going on this past month, I am going to be Vanna White to your Pat Sajak. You will do most of the talking, and I will just stand there and smile."

Baltimore is sunny and sixty degrees but incredibly windy. (Isn't Chicago supposed to be the Windy City?) I had an early Sunday morning flight, so I have pretty much the entire day to explore the city on foot. But in the harbor, flags fly at a stiff ninety-degree angle. With the gale force winds, I'm looking for shops or restaurants or museums—anything to be able to duck inside. I do a little shopping then decide to check out the National Aquarium. I wait in a long line of families with young children and international tourist groups speaking a myriad of languages to purchase my single ticket. The nice young man behind the counter says, "Just you?" Yep, just me. It turns out to be quite relaxing, an escape into the underwater world for a couple of hours.

Afterward, I realize I'm getting very hungry, and although I so much appreciate the remarkable beauty of those many colorful and varied fish, now I am suddenly in the mood for seafood. Then I think, *Hey, my appetite is coming back!* That's good! And here I am in Charm City, known for amazing crab. I decide that I am really going to splurge on dinner. But first, I should check out the exercise facilities at this hotel I'm staying at. There's a pretty fancy gym, the Maryland Athletic Club (or MAC), attached to the second floor of the hotel. I go back to my room to change into workout gear; I haven't really thought about my recent ordeal for the entire day, thanks to these welcome distractions.

But after I pull on black spandex bike shorts and a bright-blue running tank, I turn to the full-length hotel mirror, and I let out a little gasp. This top, I haven't put it on since before surgery. It's one of those strappy, sort of bare exercise tanks with a T-back and wide armholes designed to keep you cool; it has an attached inner shelf bra, and that's why I thought it might work. But seeing it on me now, I realize that my mastectomy scar extends well beyond the border of the right armhole. I stare at it in the mirror for a while. There is still quite a bit of the blue-colored adhesive skin glue overlying the incision; it looks like laminated plastic. I start trying to peel some off; it clings to both my incision and my fingers and then stretches like clear silly putty or rubber cement—or worse, like a booger that you can't get shaken off your finger. The black ink markings on my skin are also still quite visible despite the fact that I am showering every other day. I lift my arm halfway up, and if I look closely enough, I can just make out these very slight dimples and divots where I presume those three lymph nodes used to reside down below. Even above the incision (well above the top edge of the tank), I can see a faint C-shaped area of induration left over from the drain.

Well, I am starting to realize that I didn't bring any other exercise clothes, not even an old T-shirt; I wanted room in my carry-on for souvenirs, and I never check luggage, not even for a week-long family vacation. I am really stuck. I decide that I guess I am just going to have to go with this. I'll make it a short workout, twenty minutes on the elliptical, since I did quite a bit of walking today anyway. I wonder if I will run into anyone from my academic meeting.

In the early days, searching on the internet, I came across some photos of women who had their mastectomy scar tattooed. Never ever in my life had I actually considered getting a tattoo until I saw those photos. Many were quite beautiful, turning a rather-ugly linear scar into a leafy vine, a spray of roses, a dragonfly, a hummingbird, and even a line of musical notes. After surgery, I started to look at these websites again with interesting names, such as P. Ink. I even began to think, *Hey, the skin over my incision is numb.* I wonder how long that will last. Much less painful to get a tattoo! However, after I show these to Paul, he lets me know in no uncertain terms that he is opposed to the idea. Sigh. I guess I will avoid unnecessary body art similar to how I opted against reconstruction—avoid unnecessary surgery. I'm going to have to get used to how this looks, whatever scar remains, after the full healing process is complete. I'll need to view this as a thing of beauty or a sign of strength or something more positive . . . eventually. For now, honestly, not so much.

So I finish the workout quickly, go back to the room, and shower. Now I am starving, and although I keep checking my phone, I realize that I've just simply got to eat something. After searching ratings and reviews online, I walk across the street to the restaurant in the Four Seasons hotel, run by a celebrity chef with restaurants in DC, Vegas, and Baltimore. There is a highly rated Maryland Blue Crab Trio on the menu. I order this, along with a local beer, a hoppy IPA. The seafood is pure bliss—the crab cake, the fried soft shell crab, the spicy crab tomato bisque. I finally get a text from Mark; he's at a brewpub with another colleague he met on the plane, and he sends me a photo of an entire flight of local craft brews sitting in front of him at the table. I laugh, and I am slightly envious of his tolerance. After half of my beer, I can already feel it. I have barely drunk alcohol in over four weeks; one IPA might be my limit.

Mark and I meet up later in the hotel lobby to review our PowerPoint and handouts. We divvy up the slides equally so that each of us has something to present. "No Vanna White," I say with a laugh, but I'm feeling more confident about the presentation now. We spend the last few minutes comparing notes about our plane flights, cab rides, and dinner experiences. I describe my afternoon visit to the National Aquarium, and I thank him again for taking initiative, submitting our work and dragging me along to this meeting. It's only day one, and because of it, I am thoroughly enjoying that feeling of getting my life back again.

Chapter 20

BALTIMORE (PART II)

"Nobody got in nobody's way
So I guess you could say it was a good day
At least a little better than the day in Baltimore."
—Prince

The morning of the first day of the conference, there are very well-appointed coach buses waiting outside the hotel to bring us over to Johns Hopkins. I'm thinking, *Wow! These tech geeks know how to roll!* Usually, I end up walking everywhere at ACP or AAMC. It turns out they are simply worried about our safety and want to discourage us from strolling to campus by ourselves. Hopkins is, well, in a very *urban* setting. Much more so than our University of Minnesota overlooking the banks of the Mississippi. We pass row houses and apartment buildings in disrepair, surrounded by chain-link fences. Sadly, there are also numerous shrines composed of balloons, flowers, and stuffed animals where I can only assume someone lost their life. I see black-and-white signs posted in windows that read, "We must stop killing each other." It's 8:00 a.m. on a Monday, and we hear sirens approaching. Surreal.

But once we are ushered into the Turner Research building on the medical center campus, we are back in our comfort zone. There is the registration booth, the name tags and lanyards, the refreshments, the freebies from the vendors, and the reading materials to distribute. I meet up with Mark, and we start scanning the agenda, trying to figure out when and where we present. He notes, "It's ninety minutes total, presenting the same fifteen-minute talk on our online module innovation to six different small groups of faculty, *and* we are supposed to leave five minutes for questions."

"Wow," I say, "This is like speed dating. I've never done it this way before." I'm used to either standing next to a poster or having a PowerPoint and a few interactive exercises for a workshop. And usually, I have lots of time, and I am in complete control. Mark had warned me about this before, but now I am seeing that this is going to be a little bit of a marathon.

We are going to spend the morning learning about a variety of online learning innovations, IT infrastructure to support medical education, and data to drive practice improvement. There is a senior clinical informatics presenter from Epic, our practice EMR. I've circled that one on the agenda; I'd like to give that man an earful. But all griping aside, the presentations are interesting, the questions and answers well informed, and I get the general sense that these are really earnest, talented people with a strong desire to improve both health care and medical education.

During the opening plenary session, I am also scanning the attendee list, and I realize, although there is a national (even international) presence, there is a lot of representation from the East Coast—Penn, Pitt, Jefferson, GW, and of course, Hopkins. Other than nearby Wisconsin, we're the only Midwest institution I can find. This is good in a way; I like interacting with educators from different regions; they often have a novel approach or a new way of thinking that we haven't considered. But I also realize that this may have an impact when it comes to our presentation. I once gave a lecture at an ACP meeting in Philadelphia in 2004. There is definitely an East Coast style of communication, which is more direct and more to the point than Minnesota nice. They also tend to ask tougher questions and probe deeper. I'm generalizing here, but I think it holds true.

Then midway through the plenary session, the dean of education at Vanderbilt is summarizing their findings after a nearly eight-year implementation of an electronic-learning platform for their entire medical school curriculum: "I am excited to discuss further and also hear about many more innovations at this meeting." In his concluding slides, he flashes up a few selected titles out of a fairly packed agenda, and in the middle of the screen is a big maroon-and-gold *M* followed by "University of Minnesota Medical School, Heather Thompson and Mark Hilliard, Online Module Production for Blended Learning Using Hybrid Web Applications." I'm staring at it, thinking, *This might be the first time in my entire life I've been mentioned in an opening plenary session.* I look over at Mark, and he has wide eyes too! Then I think, *Oh crap, we probably didn't make enough copies of our handout.* The dean moves on to the next slide, and after that, I realize, *Darn! I didn't even snap a photo of that with my mobile!* Ironically, I think, *I am so not tech-driven.*

Later, right after lunch, is our speed-dating session. I've got butterflies in my stomach as usual; I once self-prescribed propranolol right before giving a talk for performance anxiety, but it didn't do a thing. I just have to wait it out, and those butterflies usually subside once I get going. The problem this time is that, starting over every fifteen minutes with a new audience, butterflies land again. And it's challenging to convey a big idea in this short of a time frame; we're flying through the information, trying to demo the module on the screen. We answer rapid-fire questions (definitely East Coast style) and maintain composure. All the while, when I am making a point of clarification, I am thinking, did I already say this, or was it the last group? But pretty soon, I have a good vibe about this, and so does Mark. People seem really interested. I don't know if it was the plug at the plenary or what, but wouldn't you know, we ran out of handouts.

After: Huge drop in energy level. I'm drained. I honestly could have fallen asleep in the following workshop. I feel so emotionally and physically exhausted, but I really do want to pay attention. The focus is now shifting to big data and how we, as a health-care system, really need to provide patients with access to more of their own clinical data. An informed, activated, and motivated patient is going to be the best advocate for their own health care, as the literature has shown. I couldn't agree more. Listening to and pondering this, I start thinking of how I've been using (abusing?) my own chart in Epic.

When I entered my own health-care system, I now have the ability to sign onto my own chart in the EMR. At my first check-in, the clinic coordinator asks me, "Are you on MyChart?"

I'm thinking, *Of course, I am . . . on . . . my . . . chart.* I say, "No thank you," which seems to puzzle her. I wonder if this is something that's being monitored, or if I will get a call or an e-mail. But I wouldn't have to give myself permission to view my own chart, or would I?

I was upfront with my care team. I told both RN coordinators in surgery and oncology that I would be checking my own chart for test results and follow-up appointments. They seemed fine with it, saying, "I would do the same thing if I were you." I didn't read any of my physician progress notes; that seemed a little over the top and they wouldn't provide much additional information for me anyway. A progress note using an EMR template is more or less a billing and coding construct, unfortunately.

But having this all-access pass was incredibly helpful. First, I noticed appointment times would sometimes change, such as when scheduling an MRI or the follow-up with Dr. Blaes. I'd see it in Epic, add it to my Google Calendar, and not get a standard notification until a week later. I could also see the test results that were pending, not just results that were back. Again, just having that information is better than not knowing anything.

Also (another story to illustrate the point), when I first went back to my primary-care clinic outside my system, they tried to be helpful and offered to order the BRCA testing ahead of time while I was being referred to the U. I said, "Sure, why not? It will be back that much sooner." Well, drawing the blood at the laboratory that afternoon, I began to suspect this might not be the right test by the way she read off the order, the type of tube they were drawing, and the fact that I didn't sign a genetic-testing consent form. I asked about it but got vague answers. When I got a call two days later and someone left a message with the supposedly negative result, I knew something was amiss—genetic testing takes weeks, not days. I called back and played multiple phone tag (first with a front desk person, then with a medical assistant, next with a clinic RN), asking them to clarify and even read off to me exactly what result is on the screen. This was like pulling teeth. I was starting to get frustrated. I pointedly asked, "Is this really a BRCA result?

Because it does influence the clinical decision-making quite a bit, such as 'Oh, I don't know'—the entire surgical approach." This very pleasant RN reassured me that when she typed BRCA into their EMR, by golly, this was the lab order that came out, and the result was noted to be "26." None of this makes any sense to me.

Later, once that lab result was forwarded to my U chart, I can click on it. Now I can see they had somehow ordered a CA 27.29. Yes, the range is 0 to 38, and my result is 26, which technically is normal. Apparently, this is some sort of tumor marker; the significance of which is completely unknown to me. If I could have just seen the order, as I can when I am logged in myself, I could have avoided drawing a useless lab, the unnecessary expense, and the follow-up phone calls. Even someone who is not medically trained should be allowed to do a bit of cross-checking. Any woman who has just been diagnosed with breast cancer—believe me, if they have access to the internet, they will know what BRCA is. Even worse, what if I would have heard that this test was negative when that was incorrect and the real result was actually positive or vice versa? Geez, errors in health care, don't get me started. But my point is, *empower the patient.* Let them look at their orders, their test results, and even their notes. Transparency, no matter how uncomfortable, is better than what can occur otherwise.

So I'm sitting at an academic meeting in Baltimore, 1,100 miles away from home, and I am thinking about the above scenarios in my own medical care—after really only being immersed in it for just one month—and how they directly affect my point of view. I am also realizing once again how my experience as a patient will color every single aspect of my professional life going forward. It's going to become as ingrained as the other traits and skills that I bring to the table—whether it's medical knowledge, communication, or teaching. I suppose this could be true for every physician experiencing their own health issues. I am sure I am not unique in that regard. But stopping to consider the profound impact, even on a somewhat peripheral issue we are discussing today (technology in medical education), helps me appreciate how this entire experience was, is, and hopefully always will be working toward a greater good.

Chapter 21

BALTIMORE (PART III)

"To awaken quite alone in a strange town is one of the pleasantest sensations in the world." —Freya Stark

D ay 2 of any academic meeting is generally more enjoyable and much more relaxed—unless you happen to be presenting on day 2. Luckily, I am not. That morning, I decide on a green turtleneck sweater over dark pants (mostly because it's windy, rainy, and only forty-some degrees outside), and I'd rather avoid nylons and heels. I think the weather was actually better back in Minnesota!

And the night before, thanks to sponsorship from an online board review course, we had a complimentary dinner at McCormick and Schmick's. Pretty fancy, everyone was still dressed up (suits, skirts, and dresses) and drinking either high-end wine or upscale martinis. Tonight—on Dr. Tuttle's recommendation, really and truly—Mark and I are planning just the opposite: Fells Point, belly up to the bar, eat crab legs or peel and eat shrimp with our bare hands—beer, definitely, no wine or fancy mixed drinks. So I have also dressed a little more casually for this very reason.

The conference is again quite interesting and informative. I'm going to be taking back several ideas that I could possibly implement in my second-year course. I've also exchanged business cards with a few individuals who offer to share course materials, such as lecture outlines, practice questions, video presentation, and even avatar-style simulated patients for potential use in my online modules. (I'm not really sure if this is open source or if they will be asking a steep price, but I take the information nonetheless!) All in all, it was a high-yield meeting. At the conclusion, we take the buses from Hopkins back to the hotel and go back to our rooms to ditch some of our things. Mark and I meet back in the lobby at six thirty, and given the iffy weather, we decide to take a cab to Fells Point.

As a Midwesterner, I've always been fascinated with cities that are located on either coast or the Gulf—something about seeing a large body of water next to your skyline or city view is inspiring in so many ways. Baltimore is definitely no different in that regard. Fells Point is the perfect juxtaposition of the waterfront, complete with ships large and small, some vast (apparently military) next to quaint cobblestone streets with boutique shops, restaurants, and bars. The narrow brick-row-house-style storefronts seem tiny, but most then extend way back from the street, opening up into much larger spaces than you think they would be. A city square flanked by replica gas street lamps sits in the center. The rain miraculously stops. The sun comes out for a bit; the daylight is just starting to die into dusk—the perfect lighting for taking photos. Mark and I are walking around just taking this all in. We are both fascinated by the location, the architecture, and the historic feel. I take a picture of him on the pier; he takes one of me in front of Soundgarden. We go inside this vintage music store and lose at least an hour of time; I purchase two CDs to replace in my collection those that have become hopelessly scratched over twenty years of use. In the store, I see a shrine of sorts dedicated to Prince, a reminder of how recent and how shocking his passing was. I then remember, Prince also recorded the song "Baltimore" in 2015 as a reaction to the racial tension happening there at the time; posters bearing his image are all over this area. I decide to throw in another CD, *The Very Best of Prince*, featuring seventeen of the songs I grew up with.

We attempt to get a table at Thames Oyster House, but now there is over an hour wait (which was about what we squandered in that music shop), and there were no seats at the bar. Instead, we wander back through the square, and I see Bertha's Mussels at the corner of Broadway and Lancaster, another longtime establishment. I recall reading about it earlier on another website, with pretty good ratings. I ask Mark, "How about this place?"

He replies, "I've never had mussels."

Done! That's where we are going then! I adore mussels.

We sit down. It's the perfect crowd, not at all empty but not too full either, and no loud drunks. There were a few of those, of course, out in the square; but they seemed so young, mostly guys roving around in groups, laughing and goofing around. They look barely older than Sam to me. I smile and figure that they are here for a twenty-first birthday or graduation or something—let them have a good time.

We start with the mussels steamed in Guinness with old bay and onions. Mark then orders the Shellfish Royale platter, and I order a crab cake and a half pound of shrimp. Everything is great, just fantastic. We're debriefing about the presentation from the day prior.

"That was a marathon," I say.

"But it went very well!" Mark responds. "Everyone seemed so engaged, asked great questions."

Our conversation turns from work to sharing personal stories. Mark knows about my recent diagnosis but doesn't bring it up at all unless I mention it first. He's very much a gentleman in that regard.

I say, "This trip was a much-needed mental-health break after everything I've been dealing with this past month. More enjoyable than MRIs, surgery, or doctor's appointments!"

He laughs. He then shares a story that his sister-in-law is a breast cancer survivor and relays some of what she's gone through in the past two years. "She also works at the university and chose to have her cancer care at the U as well, just like you. She set aside privacy in order to have the best treatment team." Later, he mentions her name, and I realize, *Wait, she's my patient. I've followed this entire ordeal from the very beginning. What is this, are we all just in cahoots with one another?* So many connections, it's crazy. I didn't say anything at that time though, sitting at the restaurant in Baltimore: HIPAA. And professionalism, of course. I remind myself that it's also a tacit endorsement—others, like me, have chosen to seek care in our own system despite the fact that it might be awkward. It makes me feel yet again that I made the right decision.

After finishing our seafood tour de force, Mark suggests, "It's time to check out that saloon, the Horse You Came in On."

When we enter the low-ceiling, mostly wood, dimly lit space (rowdy country bar theme—saddles as bar stools, shotguns on the wall), I say, "This reminds me so much of my small-town Minnesota upbringing rather than an East Coast hipster-style hangout!" There is a cover band, a pretty good one, but the range of music is downright mystifying—everything from Metallica to Alan Jackson to Simon and Garfunkel to the Eagles, and yes, even a bit of Prince thrown in there as a nod to current events. Mark is older than me, but I am such a bad judge of age; I can't tell how much older (maybe late fifties?). He is married, and his kids are in college, but that doesn't make it any easier to venture a guess. When we exchange notes on musical genres we enjoy and he mentions the fact that his running music is still on *cassette tapes*, then I have a much better sense of where he is coming from. Man, I thought I was bad, keeping everything on CD.

We finish our second round of beers, and I think, *I wonder if they will want to check liver function tests any time soon in preparation for starting tamoxifen.* This, on top of the wine yesterday evening, has been a pretty wild week for me. But we've also been walking around a lot and eating great food, and I am feeling good— definitely tired but more from the conference post-adrenaline crash than anything else. Still, we call it an early night and are back at the hotel a little after 11:00 p.m., fairly tame, and I sleep soundly until my usual 6:00 a.m. wake-up time.

The next morning, one last workout at that fancy gym, then shower, pack, check out, hail a cab by 8:30 a.m. for my 10:30 a.m. flight. As I board the plane, I sit in an aisle seat next to a very nice middle-aged couple in the middle and window seat. We make small talk; they are on their way back to Minnesota after their daughter graduated from medical school.

"Really!" I say. "I am an internal medicine physician. What is she going to do next?"

Her father says, "She just finished medical school at Penn, will have a transitional year at Hennepin County, followed by radiology residency at the U."

"No kidding!" I say. "That's wonderful—it's a great program!" I tell them that I now have a very special place in my heart for radiologists who train at the University of Minnesota.

Then his wife to his right mentions, "Our daughter and son-in-law have a nine-month-old baby." They show me photos on a tablet.

I think, *Ha, good for her! She's jumped in even earlier than the typical residency baby-boom time frame.*

Her father asks, "What is it like, really, being a resident? Do they get any time off, any vacation?"

I find that heartwarming; he's obviously worried about her (probably rightly so), and I tell him, "Honestly, it's not as bad as it used to be. We have duty-hour regulations now. It's a more humane training environment. The intern year is rough, but it should get much better after that. Work-life balance is possible— challenging but possible."

He seems to really appreciate that information. Both of them are listening intently to every word I am saying; I hope in some small way I am being helpful.

The flight is smooth. We land on time, no issues at all. Later I get to pick up my kids at 3:00 p.m. from school, which is a rare treat; and when we get back to the house, it's sixty-five and sunny, much nicer than the weather back in Baltimore. We hang out on the back patio, and once Paul gets home from work, I relay stories about my trip and show them pictures on my phone.

So now, tomorrow, I must go back to work after yet another stretch of time off. This is tough; I honestly wish I would've just taken medical leave up until the Baltimore trip; it would have been much easier that way as opposed to this start-and-stop business. But I'm also reflecting on how much attending this conference has benefited me physically, mentally, academically, and professionally. Good timing, I think, or should I say God's timing. I see that at almost every turn. I'm also left to ponder what else is coming my way. Not in an anxious fashion but curious— what amazing coincidence, small-world experience, or "six degrees of separation" occurrence there might be right around the corner. I've had almost too many to count in a span of about six weeks.

Chapter 22

YOU'VE GOT MAIL

Restore a man to his health, and
his purse lies open to thee.
—Robert Burton

G iven the advent of online bill paying, my home mailbox doesn't see all that much traffic; it is generally reserved for a few select medical journals, cooking magazines, and the usual junk mail. Starting about three weeks after this all began, however, it is now being flooded with a whole host of interesting items—cards, letters, appointment reminders, gift packages, test results, patient satisfaction surveys, and yes, medical bills.

First, the result letters. I find it amusing that it's the day before surgery and I open a letter that tells me I have a highly suspicious mammogram result. Thanks! I'll be sure to follow up on that! What a long lag, and I honestly wonder why we even send these things in the mail. Later, the Regions MRI report arrives. The lengthy explanation and the nature of the comments almost suggest that the radiologist is hedging, truly on the fence regarding the interpretation. I've seen this before; however, I don't envy their position, especially in my case, trying to make sense of very subtle findings in the background of extreme density. *Snowball in a blizzard.* This MRI report is followed by the biopsy report, the pre-op labs, and so on. But I notice, huh, I never got a letter in the mail regarding the mysterious CA 27.29 result somehow ordered in error when my oncologist requested BRCA testing. I suspect someone must have realized that this was the wrong test and was too embarrassed to send it.

Interspersed with these result letters (and much more enjoyable to open and read) are several cards from friends and family. The first is from Jodie, a fellow soprano in the Oratorio Society and one of my best friends. It includes kind words and a note of encouragement inside a card designed like a tree, symbolizing growth and renewal. The next is a card signed by twelve or more ladies from my women's Bible study group. I read through each one of their handwritten comments and signatures; it's very touching and heartwarming although the "get well soon" inscription on the front gives me pause. It's strange; I felt fine at that time. I technically *was* well, I guess, except for the two tiny tumors festering inside me. I have a few more cards arrive and a care package sent by my sister-in-law, Carla, and her two daughters, Josianne and Justine. This care package contains a collection of gifts obviously designed for me to pass the time, either in the hospital or at home recovering—an adult coloring book, a journal, snacks in the form of trail mix, a fancy water bottle, and a hardcover inspirational book. Later on, Lydia and I have fun with the highly detailed coloring book and the myriad of brightly colored pencils.

Also, I am now getting constant correspondence from my health insurance company. After personally avoiding doctors like the plague, having only one physical in the last three years, suddenly I have exploded onto their scene. I recall thinking, *Early on, we'll probably max out any out-of-pocket deductible. What else do we need to get done?* It turns out my husband is overdue for his first screening colonoscopy. Bingo!

But the communications coming from them are confusing to say the very least: "Explanation of benefits," "THIS IS NOT A BILL," and so on. It's also the first time when I have to commit to a somewhat large but necessary expense with absolutely no idea of what is to come. When I purchased a new vehicle in 2014, I did an amazing amount of research online prior to even setting foot at a dealership. I had my down payment, monthly payment, trade-in value of my SUV—all of this worked out ahead of time. I don't like the uncertainty of the medical bills at all.

I even tried to figure out if my own university was "in network" versus "out of network" for my particular plan and how that affected my choice of doctors and my bottom line. Despite combing through the website and reading the fine print, I am getting nowhere; I decide to call and ask the same questions over the phone.

I get a very nice, rather-young-sounding man on the other end of the line: "I am afraid the university is out of network for you." (Ah, the irony since I work there.)

I ask, "Can you help explain how that translates into real life? I would like to know the cost difference and if it is worth it to me to get the expert opinion."

He says, "Every facility or provider charges something completely different, then the payer compares the out-of-network charge to what would be charged *in* network. Next, a process occurs as to what to do with the difference, including some cost absorbed by the provider or facility and some passed on to the patient." How this is actually calculated, he cannot say despite (I will find out) the payer sending lengthy letters providing very detailed annotations/explanations: "Service not billable in facility provided." "Charge exceeds maximum allowable billable amount." I have never realized how incredibly confusing and how truly backward our system of payment is. Trying to anticipate any of the expense *before* the actual appointment (or the operation or the MRI) is next to impossible.

Finally, after all the above occurs, weeks later, an *actual* bill shows up in my mailbox. When opening this, I feel like cueing a drum roll; I am not sure if I will owe a tiny copay or a huge chunk of it. Compare and contrast: For the first MRI, almost $4,000; my responsibility, $50. I think that's a pretty good deal! For a $600 ultrasound, I owe $280. For the first office visit with surgery, $180; oncology, $360. For the same-day surgery, a total of over $18,000, and I need to pay *only $50*? But wait, that's just the facility portion, the professional fees come later—$964. None of this makes any sense to me in terms of the vast differences in what I actually end up paying. And again, it's terrible that everything is retroactive. It's after the fact, no way to plan ahead, to try to budget financially for these expenses. I have heard that medical bills are among the top three reasons that a person declares bankruptcy.

I cannot help but think about a patient of mine whom I have followed for many years, Rachel. She came to see me for a specific symptom in December of 2014. After I enter the room and greet her, she says, "I can feel a lump in my left breast. It's been there for a while, I think, but it suddenly got bigger."

I examine the area, and I have that sinking feeling; it's a very hard, irregular three-centimeter mass, easily palpable just to the left of the areola. "I have to say, I am concerned about this. Can you have a mammogram and ultrasound today?" I send her immediately to the Breast Center, and of course, the imaging is highly suggestive of malignancy. They offer to biopsy right there, but she refuses and leaves. I call her on the phone later to find out why.

"I've been having problems with my health insurance coverage. I'm wrestling with the MNsure website, experiencing technical difficulties. I need to be certain that I have coverage; I just can't afford to pay any of these expenses out of pocket." I emphasized again the suspicious finding and the need for a biopsy; Rachel says she'll come back as soon as this whole insurance thing is sorted out.

Over six months later—*six months*—she's on my schedule again. This time, it says in the EMR for a "skin rash." I walk in the room. "How are you? I haven't seen you in so long!"

She says cheerfully, "I'm ready now for my biopsy!"

I just about fainted. *This hasn't been done yet?* I tried to hide my surprise and suppress the shocked expression on my face. "Yes, let's get you in right away." And the skin rash? It turns out, the breast mass is now visible to the naked eye. Just looking at the skin overlying her left breast, I can see the irregular contours.

I was so upset by this. I spent a good half hour after her appointment searching through the EMR for documentation surrounding what happened or if we had somehow dropped the ball. There are multiple telephone notes documented end of 2014. The Breast Center had contacted her, my nurse Tony had called her, the clinic social worker as well, trying to help her navigate the financial issues. It appears that we did everything we could, short of fixing the actual problem.

As I see my own medical bills are starting to accumulate, I suddenly remember that when I received the teaching award from the medical school on April 21, it came with a $2,500 check. This was unexpected; many awards simply come with a plaque or a certificate. Just the recognition is appreciated, and it's something to list on your curriculum vitae. But as I consider this amount, I am also looking at that complicated "explanation of benefits" form, which per my read lists only one helpful figure, and that is my out-of-pocket maximum: it's . . . $2,500.

I think, *Right back at ya, University of Minnesota.* Thanks for the award; now that money is just going back into the coffers at M Health. Perfect use of it, actually, and in my opinion, another example of providence. I am blessed and truly grateful to have the extra funds in addition to the financial stability that comes with a two-income household. I almost feel embarrassed. When I think back to my patient Rachel, I can't imagine waiting six months and dealing with the fear and the anxiety surrounding it, in addition to the obvious financial stressors. I couldn't even wait six days.

I found out later that she was stage 3, HER2 positive, and would need both chemo and Herceptin. Unfortunately, she also developed a rip-roaring autoimmune hemolytic anemia from Herceptin—absolutely scared the life out of me to see her labs coming back, the plummeting hemoglobin, elevated bilirubin, and the sky-high LDH. She was admitted to the heme-onc service; the drug had to be stopped. But she's a tough lady. She survived all of this, and I am still following up with her to this day. And I cannot help but wonder if earlier diagnosis and treatment would have changed her outcomes at all. I am not sure those six months would have made any difference, but there are plenty of other instances where it could have.

As a result of the Affordable Care Act, the percent of uninsured in this country has dropped from around 18 percent to less than 10 percent. This is very good news, of course. But Rachel's story illustrates that this is only the beginning, or I should say, it's one facet of the hugely complex, multilayered, dynamic issue of providing cost-effective medical care to a population as a whole. Certainly, there is dissatisfaction on both sides of the aisle in terms of what has or has not been accomplished with health-care reform. There are still many problems, thorny issues in terms of availability of insurance plans, what coverage they actually provide, how much of the costs are passed onto the patient, the numbers of people choosing to just pay a fine rather than get coverage, then of course, the red tape, the never-ending changing of formularies, the explosion of prior authorizations, and other unintended consequences.

I realize there are no easy answers here, but at least I can honestly say, I have a much better appreciation of what it is like to be on the receiving end of medical bills. And how complex it is to navigate your own health insurance coverage, especially when a major health issue suddenly arises, and you are trying to choose your doctors to help manage it. I ended up paying more out of pocket so that I could see the surgeon and the oncologist who I thought were the best fit for me, but I realize, not everyone has that option. The same occurs with prescription drug coverage; if I am taking medication for blood pressure, and it is working great, why would I want to switch because of a formulary change? More clarity around these issues might help patients select the appropriate insurance plan. We truly need to know what we are actually getting when we sign up.

I'm also keenly aware of the high price tag on so many "routine" studies. Compared to some colleagues, even before my diagnosis, I tried to practice a bit more conservatively; I tend to order fewer tests, and rely on clinical judgement with close follow up. After this, I find I'm even more cautious, because I've seen those bills arrive in my mailbox weeks later, and have thought; was that MRI really worth it? Hopefully the influence of engaging the health care system--both in everyday practice and now my personal experience--will result in a move in the right direction, a shift of perspective, a lean towards more cost effective care.

And ultimately, I'm waiting for the day when the most medically related correspondence in my mailbox reverts to academic journals, once again.

Chapter 23

THE MENTOR (PART III)

Dearly beloved, we are gathered here today to get
through this thing called life.
—Prince

T hursday is a *Back to Work: The Sequel* and also the same
day as Charlie's surgery. I have been easing back into
work with a reduced clinic schedule, then that three-day
trip to Baltimore, and today I am up to full speed, even covering
resident's clinic again for the first time since the operation. I
had been contemplating Charlie's situation even while at Johns
Hopkins. I sent him an e-mail while I was there, telling him
all about the conference, asking him how he is feeling, how his
appointment went with oncology. He's completed all his training
in New York—medical school at SUNY, residency at Bellevue,
hematology fellowship at NYU. He very much understands the
East Coast communication style that I mention in my e-mail. He
had written back prior to my presentation: "East Coast approaches
to questioning—very direct and sometimes appear hostile usually
without that intent."

This made me feel better at the time. They won't be hostile,
just a bit more intense than Minnesota nice. It gave me the
boost of confidence that I needed to get through that marathon
presentation.

Looking ahead to my return, the morning of that Thursday, I have resident clinic; the afternoon, flexible office time. I wonder when his case is scheduled or if I would have the chance to stop by and pay a visit, maybe late afternoon. Before leaving Baltimore, I did catch up with more e-mails I was getting from both Charlie and his wife, Gay, regarding these details; it's a twelve-noon start, likely lasting three hours, and probably a two to three days' hospital stay.

"Ha!" I reply. "Captive audience! I am coming to see you whether you like it or not." At one point, he had commented on how he wasn't sure if he wanted all his colleagues knowing about this or examining the nether regions where this tumor is located or even if he would welcome visitors with his rear end propped up in the air. My reply is "If I can put up with a good portion of the university faculty staring at my chest, you can handle this." His response is "I guess now, anatomically, I will finally fulfill what they say is true—that I am doing a half-assed job." I wonder how I could apply that to me. Half-chested? Half-hearted? It doesn't work quite as well.

So that morning, there are only two residents scheduled in clinic; thank goodness, I can catch up once again with the dreaded in-basket in the EMR. I also pull up Charlie's chart just to see where he is located; it says "Admitted" and "Peri-op" in the banner, so yes, it's a go. I wonder if I will get flagged for doing that. He did give me permission to view his chart; I should probably get that in writing and scan it in.

But knowing how things work, a twelve-noon case may not start until 12:30 or 1:00 p.m. Later in the afternoon, I think he might take longer to wake up from the anesthesia. He's a bit older than me for gosh sake. If they are looking for a bed to admit him to the hospital, then they are probably calling around 5:00 p.m., which when I am on the swing shift, I have dubbed *the witching hour.* It's when the clinics are nearing the close, the ER is just starting to get busy, the patients who are failing recovery from same day surgery or endoscopy won't be able to go home, suddenly your pager is going off constantly to discuss admissions one after the other, rapid fire. Then oftentimes the patients who are being discharged from early afternoon are still occupying their hospital bed while they wait for a ride or medications to be delivered from the pharmacy or the other necessary preparations for going home. So even if a patient needs admission, we often don't have a bed immediately available, and it creates a huge backlog effect. Every time I am on triage, I think, *This is so predictable every day. Why can't we engineer systems of care that are designed around the peak flow of admissions, which is always 4:00–8:00 p.m.? If the hotels and parks at Disney can do this, moving people in and out on a much grander scale, we should be able to apply systems thinking to solve this problem!*

At any rate, I conclude that in all likelihood, I may not be able to pay him a visit until the next morning. At 5:30 p.m., I am technically done for the day, but before I head to my parking ramp, I decide to walk over past the 3C patient family lounge and down around the surgery waiting area just to see if I can find Gay. And miraculously, I spot her just as she is getting off the patient elevators on the third floor, holding dinner provisions from the cafeteria in the form of a garden salad and a fruit and yogurt parfait.

"Gay! It's Heather!" I walk over, and she gives me a big hug. She's a bit taller than me, very slender, with shoulder-length, straight, ash-blond hair and blue eyes—not a pale ice blue, something in between baby blue and slate blue. She strikes me as a very classy lady. An RN by training, she understands the medical world from being a part of it; more recently, she has dealt with her husband's previous illness (a minor stroke, followed by aortic valve replacement), then her own ordeal with appendiceal cancer in 2011, and now this most recent turn of events in Charlie's life. She's also an avid reader; I always find her with her nose in a book if she has a clinic appointment with me, and I walk in a few minutes late. Along those lines, she has also contributed as an author to several books and articles on various topics, such as ethics in nursing, coping with crisis, the patient and family dynamic.

We decide to go back to the surgery waiting area and sit down at a table where her daughter is also waiting. I get to meet Amanda for the first time; she must have Charlie's genes in terms of the looks—dark hair, brown eyes, olive skin. She chats for a few minutes but tells us she must leave very soon. I decide to stick around, to keep Gay company; I'd hate to see her sitting here all alone.

She starts with the updates. "The procedure went very well. Three lymph nodes were taken, and it was actually a smaller resection of the tumor than originally planned, with a much smaller skin graft. And importantly, no need for anything more invasive that would lead to a colostomy. Not even a drain was necessary!" I am so relieved to hear all this. No drain! Better than me! And he might even go home tomorrow. He will almost beat my record of eight hours for surgery, twenty-four hours for uncomplicated delivery.

We spend the next hour or so discussing all sorts of things. The conversation shifts from the particulars of Charlie's case to the health-care system in general, then to me. She asks, "How have you been? What's been going on? What are the next steps?"

I ask, "Did Charlie fill you in on all this?"

She says, "Well, some," so I let her in on more recent developments.

"Surgery also went well, no need for chemo, thank goodness, but I will likely start tamoxifen very soon." I tell her I have an appointment with Dr. Anne Blaes on Monday. I disclose my fears about the possible cognitive changes, the so-called brain fog on tamoxifen. She shares stories of how short-term memory changes affected her after a long illness and hospitalization, and she mentions some friends she knows with similar issues. I appreciate the insights, astute observations, the advice. For a split second, I remember I am also her doctor, then just revert right back into this new role for me, the one being on the receiving end of all the medical advice—blurred lines.

I try to shift the conversation back to Charlie since that must certainly be weighing on her mind; I decide to tell the story of how I accosted Dr. Tuttle in clinic the Friday after his biopsy report came back, to make sure he knew (a) how important Charlie was to me as a mentor and (b) how ironic it was that we were both being operated on by the same surgeon in less than two weeks while covering each other's resident clinic and teaching responsibilities. We share a good laugh about that.

She comments, "Dr. Tuttle has such a calm demeanor and so much confidence. Where does he get all that confidence? He seems so young!"

I say, "Well, he *is* the chief of surgical oncology, full professor, has over one hundred publications in PubMed. I am guessing by his years in training he is around ten years older than me." I'm saying this so she realizes that they are in very capable hands no matter how young he looks, and since I did all that research, I might as well share it! But I have to laugh; it's all relative—anyway, this whole age thing. I feel completely at ease talking with and confiding in Charlie and Gay in their seventies as I would my book club for moms, all of them thirty-somethings, of which I am probably the oldest at forty-four with kids this young. Gay also shares her positive impressions regarding Dr. Umar Choudry, the plastic surgeon; I never got to meet him, given the path that I chose.

Finally, I look up at a clock, and I realize it's after 7:00 p.m. *Wow*, I think, *I had better get going. I would guess my kids have not even been fed dinner yet.* But it's been great to chat with Gay. As I was getting up to leave, the bedside nurse from the PACU comes out to give an update; Charlie's doing great, even got up to stand and walk around already, and we are just waiting for the bed upstairs on 7C. *Good luck with that*, I think.

I am walking outside now toward my parking ramp. The campus is deserted. It's a pretty late time for me to be leaving, the sun already just starting to set, when who do I see walking toward me after crossing Washington Avenue but Todd Tuttle.

I had my phone to my ear, just about to call and order a pizza for dinner, but instead, I disconnect, take off my sunglasses, and say, "Hey!" He immediately recognizes me, walks on over, and catches me up in a big bear hug. (Much better than a Bair Hug!)

I say, "Wow, your ears must have been burning—I just left Gay Moldow up in the surgery waiting area. We were just talking about you, and I am very glad to hear everything went so well!"

We chat some more; he asks, "How are you doing back at work?"

I tell him, "Pretty good, but it's tiring." Then I mention the Baltimore trip, how great that was. I thank him again for the suggestion of Fells Point. I detail our outings while we were there; he laughs when I mention the Horse You Came in On Saloon. He tells me he's just finished having dinner at the Beacon with a graduating medical student who is off to start residency and wanted to give him a gift to thank him. I notice he is holding a gift bag in his right hand, blue-and-white-striped, tied with a blue ribbon. *Huh*, I think, *there it is, full circle, mentoring again.*

Mentoring and mentors are starting to become more significant to me than I ever could have imagined. It's more than career advice, networking, or what I think is the ultimate goal of the academic leadership—getting more publications and grants out of us. For me right now, it's about helping to navigate life and even the possibility of death. It's reaching out to people you trust when your heart is gripped by fear and anxiety. It's acting on another person's behalf even when it is outside your comfort zone or outside the usual avenues of how things are done.

Maybe I will have the chance to mentor someone in this much deeper, more significant way when I am Todd's age or Charlie's age or even right now if I look for the opportunities. It will probably mean that I will have to open up a bit more and be willing to share my personal story; that will be a change for me. Those terms "work-life balance" and "having a life outside of medicine" seem to imply that the two are separate; but I realize that, at least for me, they are inextricably linked. And privacy only goes so far when it comes to making these mentoring type connections; I'm going to have to loosen up on those reins. I'll be ready for that soon, I think.

In the morning on Friday, I stop by 7C at around 7:00 a.m., actually right after Dr. Tuttle had rounded and was exiting Charlie's room. They assigned a private room for him, thank goodness, and it's a beautiful morning, the sun streaming in from the big window with the distant view of the Mississippi River. He looks great, no different than before, sitting up in bed, leaning on his right side, of course, per the surgery team instructions. He says he has absolutely no pain. "You still probably have more pain than I do at this point!" I tease him about the fact that I had to put up with a drain, and here, he gets away without one. And again, we both agree how encouraging yesterday was, the entire operative approach and the early outcome, and yes, he will be discharged later today. Amazing!

We do chat about having surgery in general. He comments, "It affects the small everyday concerns, such as getting dressed, showering, bathing, or in my case, not being able to sit properly for quite a few weeks, three to six, depending on which surgeon I am talking to." That would be incredibly challenging, I think, for anyone. I whine a bit about not being able to run, which is really not all that limiting, but he totally gets it as a fitness enthusiast himself. I tell him I've been losing some weight; I can only assume this is muscle mass since I don't have much peripheral fat, to begin with. (And certainly, that was no eight-pound breast that was resected.) He agrees and talks about how, every time he's had surgery, it results in significant weight loss for him too. "Post-op, it's an incredibly catabolic state."

I have my own clinic starting at 8:00 a.m.; I must head over to the CSC, and so I give him a hug and tell him to say hello to Gay. The next morning, a Saturday, I would get an e-mail update from them, sent to a wide circle of friends and family that things were going well. But right after that, I also had another message from Gay, sent to me personally, that was very touching.

"You were meant to be in our lives, no doubt about it. I really feel you passed your caring for Charlie on to Todd, and that affected how he viewed Charlie and operated. He saw a vital, valuable, loved person, not a seventy-seven-year-old guy with a terrible disease."

That's a great summary, in my mind, of all of the crazy, mind-boggling coincidences I've been experiencing over the past several weeks. *It was meant to be, no doubt about it.*

We are all in this together.

Chapter 24

THE FIRST RUN

Long ago, I learned to put people to bed only for as
short a time as was absolutely necessary, for they were
like a foundered horse; if they got down, it was difficult
for them to get up, and their strength ebbed away very
rapidly while in bed.
—Charles H. Mayo

The next morning, a Saturday, is also one of the nicest
weather days I can recall. The sun is shining, the birds
are chirping, and everything is very green and in bloom.
The temperature is actually quite warm, but importantly, in
Minnesota, there is no humidity yet and no bugs. After I get up
and look out the windows, then open the front door to check the
temp, I think, *Wow, what a perfect day for a run. Should I stay or
should I go?*

I've seen Dr. Tuttle twice in the past two days; I certainly could
have asked him about this, but either I forgot or subconsciously
I didn't want to hear no. Also, I tried to get information myself
online—I didn't want to impose on him if I could answer a simple
question quickly with yet another PubMed or Google Search. But
really not much luck. First, I am once again very aware that I must
be in the minority in that just about every instructional piece or
patient education handout on resuming activity is written for
women who choose reconstruction. Also, I am surprised by how
much vague information or even misinformation is out there.

There are many women posting on fairly reputable websites via blogs and other commentaries that are clearly equating their cosmetic implant surgery with a mastectomy plus immediate reconstruction. Sorry, ladies, two very different things. So after all this, I decide I'm just going to add two weeks in my mind to when I last saw Dr. Tuttle in the office, and that was May 5. I remember thinking, *Cinco de Mayo! Let's celebrate. Break out the tequila!* But darn, my appointment is at 8:30 a.m., a bit early for a margarita. Still, in the present, I decide to heck with it. Today I am going for a run.

Paul is actually gone for most of the day. He's giving an architectural tour of a few select projects to the partners at his firm. After I take the kids to swimming lessons, we get back to the house, and I rummage through the one big drawer I have in my dresser dedicated to exercise gear. In it, there is a magenta-hued running tank with the store tags still on it; I think I purchased it many months ago off the sale rack. I take it out, and lo and behold, it has the same soft bra / removable pad set up that has become my go-to as of late. It also has a bit of a higher neckline, wider straps, more coverage. I do a little switching around of the padding, put it on, look in the mirror, and smile. Perfect symmetry, no scars visible. *Nobody would guess I just had surgery!* It's all an illusion but a pretty good one at that. I pull on spandex bike shorts and lace up my Sauconys specifically designed for an underpronator.

I then tell Sam and Lydia, "I am going for a run, the inaugural post-surgery jog." Even they sit up a bit and take notice. Sam's twelve, very responsible, and we have neighbors, the Brands, to the east. We know them well. They have a big family, five children of their own, mostly teenagers now, several of which have babysat for my kids over the years. So I feel comfortable going out for a three-mile run without them as long as they keep the doors locked, and I know the Brands are at home. In the past, when they were younger, I used to have them ride their bikes alongside me as I ran. We called it our "bike-jog," and they seemed to enjoy it as long as I promised a stop by the ice-cream shop on the way home. Now, they are way too fast on their bikes; it just doesn't work.

This time, though, I think, it's my first time running in over four weeks. What if I collapse halfway around the lake? Is this too risky? I happen to notice that this new running tank top also has a handy zippered pocket off to the side for keys or maybe a phone. I put my mobile in it, which barely fits, and zip it up, just in case.

I walk down the block at a brisk pace to warm up. I am a little nervous; when I look down at my legs, calves, quads, they seem a lot thinner to me already. How unfair it is, how quickly the human body falls into disuse atrophy! All that hard work, building up your exercise tolerance and endurance and muscle tone, and it can be lost in a matter of days. Sarcopenia, deconditioning, it happens both with surgery and hospitalization for medical reasons. I think, *Here I am, young and healthy, and went home the same day of the operation.* What must happen when we admit an elderly person with pneumonia and essentially order them to lie down for four days? It's a wonder they can even get out of bed, as per the good Dr. Mayo.

There's actually a lot of research going on in this area, and I am proud to say that the University of Minnesota is a bit ahead of that curve. There is a study in our ICU right now regarding early mobilization improving outcomes, *even mobilization of patients on a ventilator.* When I saw the e-mail sent out, complete with a photo of an intubated patient standing upright, walking around, pushing a cart full of tubes and lines and wires and IV bags and a portable ventilator in front of them, I thought, *You have got to be kidding me.* What a frightening adventure that must be! And here I'm worried about this little three-mile run.

So after two blocks of brisk walking, I break into a jog. It feels . . . great! I feel really light on my feet! I guess propelling forward 110 pounds is a bit less strenuous than lugging around 120 or more. I rhythmically pump my arms with perfect timing to my stride but not too much; my breathing settles into a familiar rhythm. My right shoulder and right arm feel a bit tighter than my left, just a little stiff but not all that noticeable. I run down Hoyt, turn right on Lexington, past the golf course, past the pavilion, down to the running path around the lake. I have a huge smile on my face, even a little tear in my eye behind the sunglasses. Ah! This is so liberating! People must wonder why the big grin. I probably look like a complete idiot.

I am just thinking, *I really should have done this sooner!* when the path now merges into a combined path for both running and biking. A few yards into this and a young boy on a bike on training wheels turns abruptly to the left, directly in front of me. I have to dodge him and turn away toward my left to avoid running into him; I feel an accompanying twisting motion of my trunk and midsection as I lurch to the side. When I do this, I feel a very odd sensation in the right chest wall; it honestly feels like there is a patch of Velcro ripping apart inside of me. *Oh no, maybe this is why I was told not to run.* But it's not painful at all, just a weird sensation, a sudden tweaking, a momentary strangeness that I have never felt before. At the time, I almost felt as though I could have *heard* it. Probably my imagination.

I slow way down, barely at a trot. I keep monitoring afterward—nothing else, no pain, no tearing sensation since. I realize that the key here is going to be consistent motion, no sudden movements; I should do a better job of scanning ahead of me for this sort of thing happening again. Luckily, the combined path separates into two distinct paths about thirty yards ahead— one for the runners and dog walkers and another for everyone on wheels. I can avoid colliding with an inline skater or another child navigating a bike for the rest of my run. I pick up the pace again.

I did fairly well all the way around the lake until I am going back up the hill climb that is Lexington Parkway; this is a tough hill anyway. Previously, it would result in fairly strenuous breathing or a stitch in my side or something to that effect. This time, I start to feel an unusual, band-like tightening, starting on the right side but now encircling the entire chest. It slowly keeps building tension, squeezing, more pressure, definitely limiting my ability to take a deep breath. Tight, tighter, tightest. Then it starts radiating down the right arm (not the left, thank God). I feel fine, otherwise, so I'm thinking, this can't be an MI. Maybe the not-quite-four-week-post-op chest wall is just not used to heaving up and down for thirty minutes straight, and it's triggering some pectoralis muscle spasm or something. I ease up, walk up the hill, and then alternate a walk/jog pattern the rest of the way home. By the time I am back to my front door, it is nearly gone. Judging by the time, though, I had a pretty fast pace up until that hill. And it feels so rewarding to have finally started down that path, to take that first step back toward presurgical-level fitness.

The next morning, I am sore as all get-out, hobbling around the house like an old woman. The quads and the hamstrings, quite tender, are noticeably affected. But the incision, not at all, I am relieved to say. And while I am, on the one hand, feeling very pleased with myself—*I did it!*—I also have a new appreciation for the healing process and what it takes for an incision or a wound to fully return to its new normal state even in a younger, healthier individual. I can also appreciate now why surgeons hate NSAIDs, heavy lifting, and crazy patients who go back to strenuous exercise too soon. I was thinking about the way it can take their wonderful handiwork and destroy it. It is sort of akin to when Paul carefully designs an addition to a 1940s cottage-style brick house in a quaint historic St. Paul neighborhood to be seamless, unnoticeable, and true to the original design, then the owners decide to raise the roof six feet or bump out the back to accomplish more square footage, ruining the entire effect.

And my final thought from this weekend outing is that I am definitely not swinging my driver again any time soon. It's made me a bit more cautious, which is probably a good thing. Maybe this is the summer I play mini golf the entire time with my kids; I'll work on my putting game.

Chapter 25

THE ONCOLOGY FOLLOW-UP

In nothing do men more nearly approach the gods than
in giving health to men.
— Cicero

The 23rd of May is a Monday. Dr. Anne Blaes has added me on to her schedule at 5:00 p.m. I can see in the EMR, it's an overbook. That warms my heart just a bit; she might be doing that to make it easier on me. I can come at the end of the day after finishing up whatever I'm doing, maybe seeing patients; I have a full schedule of my own that week. On the other hand, I feel bad about the fact that I am adding to her already long afternoon. I hope at least in part it's because she thinks it will be a quick visit, not that much to talk about; everything is going so well.

I check in around 4:40 p.m. and sit in the Masonic Cancer Clinic waiting area. This time of day, it is quite busy. I actually have a hard time finding a seat. Probably because many patients and families have been there most of the day, more and more people congregate in that space, waiting for their appointment or for a lab test or something else to return. All around me, I am reminded of what it is truly like to deal with cancer—a humbling experience, to say the least. I notice more than a few stressed patients strolling through the lobby, talking on their mobile, "The doctor says I will need another CT, and based on the scans, it's either surgery or chemo . . ." I can hear every word. In fact, it seems to amplify and echo throughout that stark modern space—I start to question this open lobby concept. I notice the patients without hair or with the elaborate headscarves. Many are wearing respiratory masks to prevent exposure to infection. It's an unusually warm day for May, and a young woman across from me is wearing a pale-green camisole with thin straps; I can see her port in the right chest wall. I get out my tablet to do a bit of work. There's another young couple to my left. He's completely bald, mask in place. He's doing the same thing, looking at his laptop, and he's telling his wife, "There is nothing like grading papers while getting chemo. It's the perfect time to do it."

A medical assistant is strolling through the lobby waiting area, calling several times for a Jennifer. She reaches the end of the hallway, turns around, stops by my chair, and says, "Are you Jennifer?"

"No," I tell her, and I look down at my locator badge clipped to the top of my shirt and think, *Are these things not working?* It would be nice if they didn't have to shout out your name, even just your first name, all over the place unless absolutely necessary. Whenever I check in here at this new building for anything now (MRI, lab, appointment), I say nothing but simply flash my badge. It works very, very well. The coordinator can see my name and look me up in the system. I think because it says "DOCTOR" in big letters across the bottom, they usually look up at me. I simply nod silently, and then they seem to get the fact that *I don't want to chat. Let's keep this on the down low. I'm looking for a little bit of privacy here, thank you very much.* Usually, they just wordlessly point me in the direction of my next stop. I am glad I figured that out, but on the other hand, I feel for the patients who have not. They could just as easily do this with a driver's license.

So a few more minutes and a little after 5:00 p.m., a nice young lady in maroon scrubs comes out and greets me, "Are you Heather?" and then leads me all the way back to the vital-signs area. I can tell she's in a very big hurry. As we are walking through the lobby again, people left and right, she's asking me, "Any pain?"

"No."

"Do you feel safe at home?"

You have got to be kidding me. In the middle of an open lobby, everyone within earshot, do you think I am going to suddenly volunteer, "Well, I forgot to mention, my husband is beating me." I am again amazed by the implications of how this new building was designed or workarounds being used as a result of it. I simply shake my head, and I give her a little "look" of disapproval, the one I often give to my kids, but it is lost on her. I'm probably the last patient of the day, and she just wants to go home. I don't blame her for that, actually; believe me, I certainly know what it's like to run out of gas after a long clinic day.

I have all day clinic every Friday, and Friday afternoon in primary care is like frontier medicine. It's the Wild Wild West. Or a full moon every week. You never know what you are going to get. It's right before the weekend. Everyone wants to be seen to make sure something is not "serious." And the other big factor, we call it "the dog ate my Percocet" phenomenon—everyone wanting their narcotics or trying to get an early refill for a myriad of reasons. I was once almost assaulted (I kid you not) on a Friday afternoon by a woman (yes, a woman) that I refused to provide any more oxycodone. After she started swinging, I stepped outside, slammed the door, leaned up against it, shouted, "Call security!" while I can hear her swearing in the room behind me. In minutes, they were there, and they dragged this woman, kicking and screaming the entire way out of clinic 3C, through the waiting room, out of the clinic entrance, and into the escalator lobby of Phillips-Wangensteen building. The real kicker? I was about eight months pregnant with Sam, waddling around, huge belly in front of a tiny frame. Maybe that triggered something in this patient; I have no idea, but needless to say, I never saw her again.

So comparatively speaking, these folks in oncology have to deal with a lot, too, but I am not sure it approaches the general craziness that is primary care. Still, even in the vital-signs area, I notice the rush-rush feeling coming from the rooming assistant. She's taking my blood pressure and my temp and my oxygen sats all at the same time. Oh well, turns out everything is normal, so I guess it's okay. And hey, if my blood pressure is 130/80 at the doctor's office, then I know it is more like 110/70 at home, so I'm pretty happy with that result after cutting the dose of my medication in half. But one concern is that when they weigh me, it's 109. *What?* I haven't weighed this little since, gosh, junior high or something. The first five pounds, yeah, that was great, skinny jeans and all; but now I've lost over fifteen pounds since this diagnosis. I think I should mention it to Anne.

I am now in the exam room. After a short wait, there's a knock, and in walks Dr. Blaes. I am not sure what it is, but the dynamic has definitely changed. She's got a big smile on her face, and those ice-blue eyes seem to sparkle and twinkle to me now. I am happy to finally see her again too. In some ways, I think, *I must be an oncologist's dream with all the good results that have returned since the first time we met.* I do appreciate, for them, how many times it's really *not* good results; the whole "breaking bad news" bit must be employed here on a daily, even hourly, basis. So let's celebrate when there *is* the return of that encouraging report. Let's all break into a song—oh wait, that's my own personal approach to be saved for the basement of my home, not here for God's sake.

I also think back for just a second to the first appointment with her and how it's sure not easy taking care of a physician as a patient. I know this quite well myself. It's very intimidating; as if your job is not stressful enough, suddenly you are dealing a patient armed with more information than you ever thought possible, someone who is possibly scrutinizing your every move, who maybe, just maybe, knows even more than you about a certain condition. Very unnerving. *What if you miss something?* I recall when I visited my local primary care clinic, prior to being referred to the U; this was the encounter where the doctor confirmed the lump and sent me off for the mammogram, ultrasound, and biopsy. She's a rather young family medicine physician, I think just out of residency. I sensed a good deal of fear on her part when she was talking with me, taking a history, then palpating the lump, then entering orders into Epic. She seemed overall a bit flustered. Later, when she called me on the phone to deliver the bad news, I told her I was thinking about transferring all my care to the U. "That's great! *Wow.* What a good idea! I'm putting in the referral right now!" I had a strong sense that she was relieved to get rid of me, but I don't blame her honestly. A physician with a new cancer diagnosis is like a hot potato. You want to pass that off as soon as possible.

But Dr. Blaes, on the other hand, seems happy to see me today. She's asking, "How have you been?" And I tell her, "Really good!" We chat about my rapid post-op recovery and the fact that I even went running for the first time this past weekend. She asks me, "How is your right arm, your shoulder?" I tell her I do notice some tightening, a decrease in the range of motion, but it's not terrible. She has me demonstrate, reaching out my right hand and extending my right arm, and then the real challenge, abduction and external rotation. She gives me some home exercises to help, then offers a PT referral if I am interested.

Next, we turn to the bigger issues. Even though all my results are encouraging, what should the next steps be? I also ask her if it's okay in her mind that they only ran the Oncotype assay on the one tumor, not both. That's been bugging me for weeks. If the one cancer has an Oncotype score of 4, great, but what if the other one is 80? She explains that the Oncotype was done to evaluate the invasive ductal carcinoma, which is the more aggressive of the two types; and if this was low risk, then the other one is likely as well. Also, lobular tends to respond well to endocrine therapy as the mainstay of treatment. After considering this, I think it sounds reasonable; I am okay with that. And that brings us to our next topic: tamoxifen.

I tell her my theory about the fact that I probably have high circulating levels of estrogen based on the migraines and other phenomena that I described earlier. I also mention my concerns about side effects. She starts to list the most common side effects: hot flashes, fatigue, skin and hair changes, weight gain. Sounds just like menopause to me. I then mention, "Hey, weight gain is not necessarily a bad thing. I've lost fifteen pounds since this diagnosis." I explained that at least five of that was pre-surgery, likely increased stress, not eating; but now I am much less anxious, back to eating normally. In fact, I ate a ton of great food while in Baltimore for a conference! She then asks, "What were you doing in Baltimore?"

I explained to her in a brief synopsis about the MedBiquitous meeting and how it was directly related to the hematology course that she helped codirect with me, initially, then handed over the reins. "You are doing such a great job with the course," she says.

That comment means a lot to me; for a moment, I am thinking not about tamoxifen but right back to academic medicine again.

Her saying that is a very high compliment coming from a practicing hematologist to a general internist for a number of reasons; first, this course is really the flagship pathophysiology course in the second year of medical school. It's been highly rated by the students for many years, and we can see by their performance on step 1 that it has been effective. The hematology course was initially developed in the early 1980s by some of our most outstanding educators in that field, including Dr. Greg Vercellotti, former dean, and my first attending on the Med 1 clerkship, and also Dr. Wesley Miller, who was my faculty advisor as a medical student, then end of intern year recommended me for chief resident, and just prior to graduation hired me as gen med division director, and later served as my department chair until 2013.

So to allow that course to be taken over by another educator, who is a generalist and has no specific training via fellowship in hematology could almost be viewed as a risk. But because these amazing faculty all seemed to believe in me, I tried to rise to that occasion, even volunteering to present a large group lecture on anemia and also assigning myself to a hematology small group. I've had to explain some very tough concepts in that small group, such as sickle cell anemia, thalassemia, thrombotic thrombocytopenic purpura, and the like; the first year was challenging. Since then, it's become easier. The material is very engaging, and I enjoy it immensely; my teaching evaluations seem to reflect that. I often tell students after filming an intro for one of my online modules that I'm not a hematologist but I play one on TV.

I cannot help but wonder now about this course director assignment that was given to me years ago. I had been working closely with Anne at that time to ensure a smooth transition. Now she's my doctor; she's my oncologist. Could this be the real reason behind it all along? To start to merge our paths? To prepare me for such a time as this?

Back to the tamoxifen question. I do mention to her my fear about cognitive dysfunction. She reminds me, "You have to be careful what you are reading because many of the studies regarding tamoxifen are also in patients who have received chemotherapy. So it's going to be difficult to tease out what is what in terms of the effect." I appreciate that information; everyone in this field has heard of chemo brain, which could make some sense. If these drugs target and kill rapidly dividing cancer cells, it seems plausible that they could target cells in the neurological system. Anyway, I am somewhat reassured. Even so, I ask her if it is okay if I wait to start the tamoxifen after my inpatient attending in June just to avoid the onset of any potential side effects during a very busy and stressful week. She agrees; that would be just fine. I neglected to ask about the sexual side effects, if she sees that very often in her practice. Here I am, a physician by training, and I am too embarrassed to mention it. Instead, I just think to myself, *I am still hoarding that box of Vagifem samples if need be.*

Now it's on to the physical exam. She wants to feel my lymph nodes and inspect my incision and my right arm. She does a very thorough exam, quite prolonged, lots of pushing and prodding, and I appreciate that because her first response, seeing my exposed chest, was "Wow! The incision looks great!"

I tell her, "Beats me! It would have to be spewing pus for me to know something was going on!" She has a good laugh. I even tell her that in the early post-op state, there was so much soft-tissue swelling that when I looked in the mirror, my right "breast" appeared about the same size as it was before, and I felt like sending a text to Dr. Tuttle, saying, "I think you forgot something here." Again, she bursts out laughing. "You are so funny with your comments! You should keep up that sense of humor. It's a good approach."

We chat a bit about the follow-up going forward, and she says I can always e-mail her with a note about how I'm tolerating tamoxifen or if I have any other questions. We're also anticipating what should happen with the imaging. I remind her again of the long, drawn-out MRI saga; she says she'll have a chat with our breast-imaging team and come up with a plan. All I am thinking is, never order an MRI the week before my cycle—that much I know. Although something funny happened in Baltimore. I had a surprise visit from Mother Nature in that regard, and there was no early warning sign for me, which was usually pain in the left breast. I had to run out at night and find the nearest CVS, which was annoying. I thought, *Huh, I wonder what that was about.* Maybe the left one was saying, "Gee, what happened to the right one? I better remain very quiet over here, or pretty soon I'm going to have a surgeon standing over me with a scalpel in hand."

But overall, it's been a very good visit with Dr. Blaes. I tell her, "I'll keep an eye on my weight. I will continue adding in some protein shakes." She wants to check some baseline labs. Since it's getting late in the day, I ask if I can come back tomorrow. Another seemingly small but to me significant advantage of seeking care right here on campus is that I'm always around, and I can easily come back to get things done.

I exit the clinic, out past all those people in the waiting area, down the winding staircase, and leave the CSC. I decide to walk outside since it's a warm and sunny day, back to my Washington Avenue parking ramp. All the while, I'm replaying that visit in my mind, and other than the awkward time in the lobby space, it was a very productive, useful, and encouraging appointment. I am feeling confident once again that I am in excellent hands. I start to think, *Hey, I could become the poster child for M Health.* And at that point in time, the old Hair Club for Men commercial pops into my mind from the mid-eighties: "I'm not only the president, I'm also a client!" A very old advertising slogan but obviously effective as it still came to mind after all these years.

Well, I'm not only a doctor here; I'm also a patient.

Chapter 26

THE MENTOR (PART IV)

The sooner the patient can be removed from the
depressing influence of general hospital life, the more
rapid their convalescence.
—Charles H. Mayo

The Friday prior to my Monday oncology appointment, Charlie was sent home after a brief overnight stay in the hospital. I knew he was looking forward to going home, just as much as I was when I realized my operation would also be a same-day procedure. At times, I have a hard time understanding, even now, why some patients are so reluctant to be discharged. I could tell story after story on the inpatient medicine service of the great lengths we must go to convince some patients that it is time to leave. They are medically ready. We are comfortable with the discharge plan. There is nothing we are doing here that you cannot do at home. You are potentially exposing yourself to C. Diff, MRSA, thrombotic risk—the list goes on. At times, I think we could say, "There has been a bomb threat called in, and everyone who is medically stable must evacuate immediately." We'd hear, "But I am due for my next scheduled Dilaudid at 2:00 p.m., and I just ordered a lunch tray from the food service. I am not leaving until I try the beef stroganoff."

On the other hand, the main problem with early discharge is what could happen next at home. I recall that night when I woke up with new onset pain and had to perform my own "cross cover" evaluation. Thankfully, it worked out just fine, but obviously, I'm medically trained—what about the patients who are not? Or I would even argue that as physicians we all have areas outside of our expertise, things that are challenging to evaluate. In my clinic, as a female physician, I tend to acquire more female patients. Last time I looked at my panel, it was 70–80 percent women or something like that. So I get less and less comfortable over time evaluating problems or symptoms I hardly ever see. If I get a middle-aged man on my schedule with testicular pain, I panic. I seek a second opinion from Charlie or from Jim Langland or have to pull up a review in Up to Date. Also, patients have a very hard time realizing what a general internist can or cannot do. I love the variety. I enjoy all aspects of medicine, but there is often a look of surprise when I tell them I don't do endometrial biopsies or that the workup of hematuria in a renal transplant patient requires multiple subspecialists to get involved. I think the craziest thing I ever did in the PCC was a large volume paracentesis on a Friday afternoon when it just needed to be done, and I couldn't get the patient scheduled with interventional radiology. My resident, Mithun, and Ann, my nurse, were very supportive of the idea; but still, everyone was rather surprised seeing eight 1L evacuated bottles exiting that room and also concerned about the fact that her blood pressure was 90/50 afterward—but that's pretty normal for a cirrhotic.

The point being, there is a time and place for everything, and there are limits to our medical knowledge base and skill sets, which brings me back to Charlie's case. Two days after discharge, he is at home. He can't sit down, and he must stand or lie on his side (that is certainly stressful enough as it is), and he develops a lot of swelling and some bruising. Also, unlike me, he's on Coumadin, that wonder drug that complicates everything, especially in this type of situation. He's getting worried, and I know that must be the case when he and his wife, Gay, send me a question via e-mail, complete with an attached photo of the entire postsurgical area, including the newly formed flap, suture lines, staples, apologizing all the while but asking, *What do you think? Is this normal?* I am staring at this image at home on my tablet device, even rotating it and tilting my head to the side to try to get a better sense of the anatomic orientation. And actually, I think it looks pretty good but definitely has much more in the way of ecchymosis compared to my incision. Isn't this crazy? Shows how little we internists know about wound healing when I am comparing his surgical site to mine and trying to make a judgment call—completely different operations, different anatomic locations, different background medical issues.

I write back to him: "I think it looks good for POD 2!" But I also mention that they could phone the number we call Fairview Direct, 612-672-7575, and ask to speak with the surgery resident on call. Or come to think of it, why not send that same digital photo to someone who actually knows what they are looking at? I'm now thinking back to the conference in Baltimore regarding the use of technology in medicine. This is a perfect example of how Skype or Facetime or just simply sending a photo could quickly solve a problem, get an answer to a question without even having to make that clinic appointment, drive to the hospital, or God forbid, spend six hours waiting in the ER on a Saturday to accomplish the same thing. Why have we not been encouraged to utilize this more? I wonder. It probably has to do either with liability or with the inability to capture revenue with these type of encounters. But if the system is going to continue to push for more outpatient care because it is safer, less costly, and so on, then we had better start designing more efficient ways to access your doctors from home.

It's not quite the same, but I have always, from day one, put my e-mail address on my business card. Years before I actually had to dial the call center myself as a patient, I realized this system of phoning our office and trying to get in touch with a real, live human being is simply broken. It turns out that a patient could get my e-mail address if they really wanted to from the University of Minnesota website anyway. And I think there is a huge placebo effect with that business card. Just having my e-mail as an alternate contact brings my patient a sense of security. I have only a handful of patients who e-mail me regularly, and it's always for a good reason; they need to send me a quick update in a complicated situation, or they tried to call and didn't get through, or they are about to run out of medication and need to expedite the process for a refill. My patients have never, in over ten years, abused it. I've also never gotten an e-mail stating, "I'm having crushing substernal chest pain radiating down the left arm," on a Sunday night, which is probably what that whole liability issue is about. I think back to my own situation, having the ability to send a text message to Dr. Tuttle, that was extremely helpful. Hopefully, I didn't go over the top in some of my panic moments, but it is another example of how our systems of care really need a major redesign to catch up with technology.

But interestingly, at the end of the day, Charlie contacts Dr. Jim Langland, his primary MD; and instead, he pays them a visit at their home on his bike. Wow! Talk about the antithesis of technology—*a house call!* Throwback, retro, old school, but also what a huge relief for Charlie not having to phone the clinic, schedule an appointment, then get into the car and sit sideways and endure the ride into the CSC and the whole parking/check-in/rooming, finally get a doc to actually look at the wound and deliver an opinion, and then start the entire process in reverse. How good of Dr. Langland to go the extra mile, literally and figuratively. It turns out, he agrees with me; he thinks it looks fine. At least we have two general internists now thinking the same thing. Safety in numbers. Charlie has a follow-up with surgery but not until the week after.

Over the coming days, I get several e-mail updates from both Charlie and Gay, and on Wednesday morning, he alludes to another potential source of anxiety: the pathology report. He writes: "I have not looked up my path report yet in Epic, not sure it will make any difference knowing or not knowing until I see oncology."

What? I sure as heck know that knowing or not knowing makes a big difference from a mental health perspective. I recall reviewing my own path report in the basement on my home computer on a Sunday evening, not being able to wait even one more day. I see this e-mail and do the countdown in my head as to what date the surgery was performed and when the pathology should be back. It's been five days, including the weekend; that should be enough time by now to take a look. But I am not sure if I should do this myself again, not knowing if I am breaking any rules by accessing his chart. I decide to wait until I get to clinic and I can talk to Dr. Langland about it.

In the collaboration zone in the PCC, I am typing away at my charts from the morning when Dr. Langland arrives for afternoon clinic. It's actually a *very late* afternoon clinic; in the new building, we now have these 3:00–7:00 p.m. blocks of clinic time to be able to offer extended hours to the patients. However, I had to boycott this four-hour block personally because my schedule depends heavily on a nanny who will not want to work until 7:00 or 8:00 p.m. unless I significantly increase her pay. That being said, there are several physicians in our group who do not mind this 3:00–7:00 p.m. block; one is Dr. Langland, whose children are all grown and flown out of the nest, and also some of the newer docs who are not yet married or have kids of their own. I'm really stuck in the middle. I'm holding out until someone tells me I *must* fill an evening clinic or a Saturday morning to maintain my faculty position.

So I mention to him about Charlie: "I think the path report should be back by now."

"Oh! That's right! Let's look it up!" he says. He is sitting at his workstation, and I am standing behind him; he is extremely tall, and I am peeking over his shoulder, craning my neck, trying to look at the screen in Epic.

Here is what we see:

Final diagnosis:
A. Left femoral sentinel lymph node #1, excision:
- One lymph node, negative for metastasis (0/1)

B. Left femoral sentinel lymph node #2, excision:
- One lymph node, negative for metastasis (0/1)

C. Left femoral sentinel lymph node #3, excision:
- Two lymph nodes, negative for metastasis (0/2)

D. Soft tissue excision:
- Skin and subcutaneous tissue with previous surgical site changes
- No evidence of residual carcinoma

Three negative lymph nodes and negative surgical margins—*sound familiar?* This is so similar to my own path report; I can hardly believe it. I let out a squeal and clap my hands across my mouth; Langland looks at me like I have lost my mind. But he doesn't know about my situation. He is not yet privy to that information. Of course, he knows about Charlie, but he has no idea about all of the connections and coincidences leading up to this. I don't think he understands how much this result means to *me* or *why*, given my recent ordeal. So I try to explain away my reaction: "Well, you know him. He's been waiting for this report, probably feeling anxious. He's been e-mailing me multiple times a day, and I am pretty sure he is not aware of this result yet. Call him. Call him!" I'm practically shouting at this point.

So Langland calls and unfortunately gets routed right to voice mail. He starts mumbling his voice mail message into the phone. I open my e-mail on the computer next to him and type the following to Charlie:

Subject: your path report!!! :-)
GREAT NEWS . . .
You need to answer your phone, Langland is calling! We're sitting here in front of Epic.
All three of your nodes are negative and no residual tumor in the soft tissue. I am almost in tears; I am so happy!

The first reply was from Gay:
We were resting and now I'm jumping for joy!!!!
Such great news.
He was out walking Biscuit I must have called him 10 times before I finally got him :-)
Thank you both so much for everything.
G

Right after that, I sent a text to Dr. Todd Tuttle: "Charlie's path report: amazing!"

He texts back: "I know!"

And I'm sitting in the collaboration zone, a big smile on my face, thinking, *Wow, who could have predicted such an incredibly great outcome? Times two.* A few minutes later, Charlie also replies to my original e-mail in his usual brief, cryptic, truncated sentence response:

> i sort of figured with you all worrying
> i did not have to
> thanks so much
> you know me and my phone aversion

Chapter 27

TONY APPRECIATION DAY

Constant attention by a good nurse may be just as
important as a major operation by a surgeon.
—Dag Hammarskjold

T he end of May is a very nice time of year in Minnesota;
the weather is finally turning from spring-ish to warmer,
a nod to summer just around the corner, although now I
already have to swat at a mosquito one evening sitting out on the
patio. There are graduation ceremonies of all kinds happening on
campus. From the undergraduate programs to the law school to
the medical school commencement, there are lots of celebrating
going on. End of May is also an important milestone for me and
Dr. Jim Langland in the Primary Care Center. It's the anniversary
of the start date for our nurse Tony Frisk.

Over the years, our clinic has seen a lot of turnover of nursing
staff. From 2002 to 2010, I had been assigned four different RNs,
basically a new nurse every two years. This is challenging to say
the least; we need to get to know each other's practice styles, the
particulars of my patient panel, the way to help each other "get
things done" for the patients while in clinic but also in between
office visits. This turnover meant that, just as soon as we were
done establishing rapport and getting a good rhythm with the
workflow, I'd get an e-mail that so and so was leaving the PCC
for greener pastures. I began to think, *Is it me? Am I really just*

a bear to work with? Are my patients driving them crazy? But no, it
was happening throughout the clinic, to other providers as well.
I recall one of my former nurses became a trainer for Epic, one
became a research coordinator, another went over to cardiology,
and one decided ENT was more interesting. Primary care, it's just
tough. You must deal with anything and everything. There's a lot
of paperwork, forms and things that get sent our way. There's the
entire business of narcotic refills as mentioned earlier. And the
phone calls, phone triage—it can be anything from "My husband
seems ill, he's really confused, he's not making any sense" to "I
never heard back about my cholesterol result." As an RN, you
have to know a bit about everything and decide when to respond
quickly. It is not for the faint of heart.

So when Tony arrived in 2011, he was assigned to the Gold
Team. In the mid-2000s, as our primary care practice grew to well
over twenty providers, we needed a way to get organized; and
we decided to form three teams—Gold, Silver, and Maroon—after
the University of Minnesota colors. Each team was comprised of
seven or more doctors, a nurse practitioner, three or four medical
assistants, and two RNs. It's a great concept—rather than working
within a large rotation of random different people, we get to know
each other within a smaller group, and more importantly, we are
all located in the same team room, the same physical space. It's
amazing how much this co-localization facilitates collaboration.
In between patients, Tony would lean over to me and say, "Oh,
by the way, your patient Judy, she fell and broke her hip and was
admitted yesterday," or "I got a call from Laura. She's not doing
well. She's having abdominal pain again. She's on your schedule
for Thursday morning." Or I'll mention to him about an abnormal
chest X-ray finding that needs a follow-up CT scan. This verbal
communication simply cannot be replaced by electronic messages
in Epic.

After my maternity leave in 2007, upon my return, I was
reassigned from the Silver Team to the Gold Team to better balance
out the number of providers (and it might have had something to
do with another RN leaving). The Gold Team MDs also included
Dr. Sharon Allen, Dr. Susan Diem, Dr. Jim Langland, Dr. Charles
Moldow; this definitely played a large role in allowing those
mentoring relationships to be fostered. I recall more than once

that I had to bring my kids to work because my childcare fell through. I've actually staffed resident clinic with Sam playing games on the computer and Lydia coloring in a coloring book or listening to Adele on Tony's phone. One Friday afternoon, Sam asked Dr. Langland, "Why is this called the Gold Team? Are they ranked?" We all joined in a hearty laugh at that one. Langland then says in his big booming voice, "Yes, Sam, they *are* ranked, and your Mom is the captain of the Gold Team."

So the Gold Team is obviously very supportive of one another, and Dr. Langland and I have thoroughly enjoyed working with Tony ever since his start in 2011. He's a fantastic RN, incredibly knowledgeable and skilled, and at the same time, very practical and efficient. He really works hard and knows how to get things done. Importantly for the Gold Team, he also has a great sense of humor. His infectious laugh can be heard throughout the team room—or now I guess the touchdown space. And this is going on six years now! Quite a run for the PCC! And we decided long ago on a very good suggestion from Langland that rather than throw a party when a staff member *leaves*, we should start celebrating when they *stay*. That is the basis of the annual Tony Appreciation Day.

Langland always springs for gourmet pizza to be delivered from a local spot in Stadium Village, and I will bring dessert, usually a big pan of bars. I'm a big believer in homemade goodies; something brought from home that you made yourself is really trying to show someone you care. Last summer, when the farmer's markets at the U were bursting at the seams, I started to make pickled beets and homemade salsa using the incredibly fresh produce. Pickled beets—very Midwestern, and I love them, but what a pain. First, you roast them in the oven; then cool them; then peel them by rubbing with a paper towel; then boil the brine with cider vinegar, sugar, allspice, cinnamon, and cloves; then pour into jars. You then seal them and stick in the refrigerator for at least a week. It's labor-intensive, and my entire kitchen would be bright pink, as well as my hands. But presenting friends, neighbors, and yes, Tony with a jar of those pickled beets, that was the real reward for me. It lets them know how much they are appreciated. I am sure I got this from my Grandma Jeanette, who did the same thing with her wonderful jams and jellies, and of course, *pickled beets*. All of the Thompson clan would fight over these things at Christmas.

As I am leafing through my cookbooks, trying to decide what type of bar to bring this time around, I am thinking about how important our nurses are to providing excellent patient care. I work for University of Minnesota Physicians, recently re-named M Health. But even that former name is somewhat physician-centric. I feel from a leadership standpoint that we do not place enough emphasis on primary care, and team based care, with the correct staffing models to accomplish robust primary care in the outpatient clinic. This includes just the simple notion of hiring enough nurses to support the docs to get the work done, to keep things moving even when the physician is out. Or consider the mantra of "Right person, right job." RNs should be doing RN level work, not scheduling routine appointments or giving out normal lab results over the phone. In general, I feel we are short-staffed and our nurses are simply overworked and underappreciated.

I have encountered the importance of nurses first-hand throughout the past two months, and so has Charlie. We both have examples in our minds of where everything went smoothly, a seamless flow of care. There are also some instances where it would have been nice to have some extra help—not necessarily from the physician but from their support staff, from their nurse, or someone else who is familiar with the patient or the situation or the procedure. Consider same-day surgery or the early discharge to home. While on the one hand it's great, recovering in your own bed, on the other hand, you are also functioning as your own RN, nursing assistant, night float coverage, on-call doc. Or your spouse or significant other will be forced into that role. And it's difficult, honestly, to assess *yourself*. You are the least objective person in the world. You will either overreact, panic, wondering, *Is this normal? Is the incision supposed to look like that?* Or you will be in denial; *everything is fine* despite the fact that the area surrounding the wound is swelling to twice its normal size and draining fluid. And health-care professionals are famous for this, the denial part of it. A simple phone call to check in and see how it's going at home—that would be a great move in the right direction. It's also been shown in the medical literature to reduce readmission rates. And when a patient is at home, recovering, not feeling 100 percent, it would be nice if the phone call were initiated by the clinic team instead of the other way around.

Consider also the weekend phenomenon. Why is it that everything important seems to run up against the weekend? When I was at home and had that searing pain in the right chest that woke me up out of sleep, I thought I should maybe call and let someone know since it was a "new" symptom. On the discharge paperwork, of course, it says, "Call the doctor if X, Y, Z," followed by very generic instructions: pain, fever, drainage, and so on. So I called first thing in the morning and left a voice-mail message, of course, on a Friday. I didn't get a call back until Monday afternoon. Now granted I probably would have known enough to call again or go to the ER if the pain worsened or any new symptom presented themselves, but not every patient is this savvy. And if something bad was happening, it is probably not wise to wait until Monday.

When Charlie and Gay sent me the picture of his wound via e-mail, of course, it was a Saturday. Initially, after both my "telemedicine" assessment and Dr. Langland's house call, things seemed okay. But he was discharged on a Thursday. His follow-up appointment with surgery was not until the week *following*; this is fully twelve days since the operation, and that is just a lot of time, in my opinion, to be watching, waiting, questioning, checking, wondering, *Does this look okay?* Then after the first appointment with Dr. Choudry in surgery, Charlie has his staples removed, which is very exciting and good progress and all that; but later in the day, something happens. Something really opens up and starts draining. He's going on a walk with his dog, and his entire backside suddenly feels damp, very wet, and—*holy cow, what is going on here?*

Gay starts calling; remember, she's an RN by training and certainly knows enough to recognize something serious might be happening. She's trying to get through to the call center; I imagine she must be getting routed to various phone triage lines or having to leave voice messages as I did. I've come to find out later that it was *twenty hours* before she finally gets to speak with a real, live person on the other line. That's an entire day passing by with a minute-by-minute buildup of tension, fear, anxiety, trepidation, frustration, even anger now, added to the mix.

At the in-office visit with Dr. Tuttle the next day, Gay came prepared by writing down a list of questions. Later, she e-mails me an update. She seems overall very happy with the appointment; she writes: "I asked lots of questions today to Tuttle and kept asking till I got the answers. Tuttle's so good. We like him so much. But I wouldn't leave until I had his nurse's number, and I was feeling very pushy, but eventually, I got it." She goes on to describe the next steps. After a period of wound healing, likely radiation, possibly chemo, other decisions will have to be made. I did reply to this e-mail; I told her about my unfortunate experiences trying to get through the call center myself or leaving voice-mail messages, hoping to help her feel better. *Hey, it happens all the time.* But she responds with some incredibly insightful observations:

"I believe the job of the caregiver is harder than that of the patient. The patient needs to heal and live through the emotions of surviving the surgery and healing, granted, no small task. The caregiver though has to do the observation, reporting, supporting, cooking, pretending that life is normal, dressing changes, communicating, driving, applying stuff to the skin, etc., and has to survive the emotions of loss and grief and hope and terror at the crises that keep occurring: 'Have we done something wrong?' 'Have *I* done something wrong?' 'Will the wound open?' 'Is it infected?' 'What's happening?' When I was finally able to talk with a nurse in person, I started feeling more connected and a little more relaxed. So my battle cry is, we need nurses to take care of us and tell us what to expect, whether it's going to be good or bad. The caregiver and patient need information. We don't care good or bad, we need to know! Thank you for listening to me sound off."

Yes, indeed, *we need nurses to take care of us.* And not just as a result of my recent ordeal; I'm thinking now about Tony and how valuable his help is to me on a daily basis. I realize if he left the U, I would be right back at square one, starting over with someone new. And many of my patients, they would absolutely panic at the prospect of him leaving. I've decided that in addition to bringing treats next week, I really need to speak with the medical director of my clinic about some of the new "workflows" that were established upon the move to the new building. For over two months now, there has been a routing of all the patient phone calls that used to be covered by the call center to our pool of RNs due to staffing issues, simply not enough people to answer the phones. There needs to be some of that burden lifted as soon as possible. We can't lose great nurses because they are constantly filling in, covering some other gap in the system, stretched too thin to be able to devote time and energy to what they value most—direct patient care and interacting with their providers. I also think, the above stories truly illustrate that the most brilliant doctors in the world are nothing without their RNs to support them.

Back to the pickled beets. It's spring, and Tony has informed me that he is going to plant a garden this year, and in it, in addition to zucchini and tomatoes and watermelon, he's growing an heirloom variety of beets with the very enticing name Bull's Blood. Excellent! We make a plan. He can grow the beets and bring them into clinic 4B, and I will pickle them! What a team, I must say. Teamwork is what it is all about. Sadly, I reflect, we no longer have the Gold Team room—it's now that blasted collaboration zone, infiltrated by dozens of random people, and the RNs are sitting way back in the touchdown space, completely separated from their doctors. Who in their right mind came up with that plan? Another issue to mention to my clinic medical director is there has got to be a way to approximate the former care team model, the co-localization aspect. Maybe we can rework the adjacent areas to better facilitate communication or use some of the pods or consult rooms to pair up the RNs, docs, CMAs again. Something, anything, or we have lost what we spent years trying to perfect.

Perhaps the new name for the team should be Bull's Blood. I like it. It sounds as though we are the strong, the tough, the survivors. Hey, at least we didn't jump ship and leave the university entirely, as a few have done already as a result. It also sounds, quite frankly, like what we all need to get through a transition such as this one. As it turns out, there is also a full-bodied red wine from Hungary by the same name: Bikaver (*bika* meaning "bull," *ver* meaning "blood"). Another version from Spain, Sangre de Toro, or blood of the bull, usually a blend of Garnacha, Syrah, and Cariñena grapes. Adjusting to a new clinic building, mourning the loss of the old team space, yet trying to remain positive and optimistic about the future—all of this would benefit, in my opinion, from a good dose of red wine.

Maybe I will bring a bottle of *that* to Tony Appreciation Day.

Chapter 28

PLEASE REMAIN SEATED UNTIL THE RIDE COMES TO A COMPLETE STOP

Summer, it turns me upside down.
Summer, summer, summer.
It's like a merry-go-round.
—The Cars

I n the coming weeks, I feel a tangible slowing, a deceleration, a ritardando. The pace of the month following my initial diagnosis was so incredibly rapid; looking back, I cannot believe the amount of imaging, labs, office visits, consultations, then surgery, then recovery, then follow-up—all in a matter of four weeks. And in the middle of that, everything is happening in an eerily similar fashion to Charlie. It is a whirlwind, to say the least. When I think back to March, remembering our spring-break trip, it honestly feels like it was five years ago.

Now, it's early June. The kids are out of school. Wow, where did the time go? The weather is perfect—warm days, cooler nights. It's light outside so early now—5:30 a.m.—that I wake up due to the skylights above in the bedroom and go for early morning runs that are so peaceful. This time of year is, of course, cherished in almost every way because of our unusually long, harsh winters. But for me, it's not just the weather; I'm feeling right now that I can take a deep breath and finally, well, relax. I take note, I don't even have any pending labs or any specific future appointments scheduled for me in Epic. I can finally take a break from reviewing my own chart! I know it's a milestone of sorts when I have not clicked on my own chart (or Charlie's for that matter) for a good two or more weeks.

I also have a slowing of my mood in a good way, I guess, because I began to wonder if a person can develop bipolar this late in the game. I've had a few highs, almost hypomanic periods accompanying the sheer elation of finding out good news, complete with euphoria, slight pressure of speech, reduced need for sleep. Somebody, please, take the credit cards out of my hands; I might go on a spending spree! Then later, when I *do* realize I have no specific follow-up scheduled, I feel just a tiny bit sad, a little let down, slightly lost, when it's been such a huge part of my life for the past two months. But after a while, this low feeling also dissipates, and I level off. I am left with the new normal of me.

I am starting to feel a bit more normal physically as well. I've gained back a couple pounds, thanks to one of our favorite pastimes, grilling out on the patio—steaks and burgers to the rescue. Running, thankfully, comes back quite easily too; I think some of the weight might actually be muscle. But there is one real setback—Sam is very much into basketball, and now, following his lead, Lydia's a pretty decent shot too. Memorial Day, the first time I venture out and shoot hoops with them at a nearby park, I go in for a right-handed layup, and let out a yell and nearly fall to the ground while the ball barely makes contact with the backboard. "What? *What?*" Sam shouts. "My arm!" I groan. "Your mom is hobbled! Unfair advantage!" I realize that it was not good. I can't raise my right arm. I've really got to get on the ball with home physical therapy. How will I ever swing a golf club? Later, back at the house, I immediately go to the internet, looking up some exercises, such as walking the wall and so on. These simple maneuvers do have some benefit, but I definitely still have a limitation in that right arm. I contemplate calling Anne about a PT referral.

Although actually, when it comes to using the words *normal* and *physical* in the same sentence, I have to admit I have a long way to go. It's still a work in progress. I recall the first time I used the locker room at my gym, with quite open public areas for changing and showering and so on. I'm in my own little world, lost in thought, trying to change out of work clothes into exercise gear when suddenly I remember, *OMG!* I am going to scare the heck out of any fellow faculty or students who are here to use the university rec center and happen to glance over my way at just the wrong time. I quickly try to cover up with a standard gym-issued yellow towel, which is about the size of a postage stamp. I can barely wrap it completely around my body to give an adequate amount of coverage for my current problem, which is sad considering I'm not a large person. Later, after the workout, the same thing in reverse, getting undressed. I'm standing there, tiny towel as a cover-up, furtively glancing around. Then I grab my tote with the shampoo and shower gel and practically run the full length of the locker room into the area with the shower stalls that now actually have curtains. I start to think, I've simply got to bring a bathrobe to the gym now or at least one of those very large bath towels with the Velcro across the top so I can wear it like a wrap or a toga. Just like in college.

Also, as we transition from late Minnesota spring (which could mean forty degrees and rainy) to now this warmer period in June, I am reminded of the continual adjustment that occurs after a mastectomy even just in terms of wardrobe options. What will I do with this strapless sundress? The whole athletic bra thing, well, that just won't work; into the donation box it goes. Same with the T-back tank tops with the cutaway ruffles. It's summer— what about my favorite swimsuits? Oh, dear. I really don't want to go swimsuit shopping again, especially in this current state. I get out my sewing kit; I take a look at some of those foam pads I've taken out of the athletic bras. I'll probably put my sewing skills to use once again and create my own answer to the wardrobe malfunction.

I am also reminded that our thirteenth wedding anniversary, ironically the very same date as my surgery, was supposed to be remembered with the traditional gift of lace. Lace really means only one thing to me in that context, and that's some sort of fancy lingerie. Needless to say, it simply just didn't happen. I think Paul had no idea what to shop for, given my new anatomy, which is understandable. It's the very first time I didn't receive a "traditional" anniversary gift, and yes, leather, stainless steel, paper, pottery—*everything else* has made it into the rotation. For a while, I feel sad, even a bit angry, that surgery takes that away from me. But then later on, I pause to consider the alternative—metastatic breast cancer? I guess I am fine, really, with going back to the old standby—flowers and chocolates. And in addition to that, I get a very nice anniversary card the next day from Paul, with an inscription proving he knows me very well. Inside he writes, "Sorry this is a day late. I wanted to make sure you were still around." Reading this card, I laugh out loud. Now *that* shows he appreciates my sense of humor.

Speaking of surgery, I have another really surprising finding: a few people, and not just one, ask me when is my next upcoming operation. At first, I pause, not even realizing what they are asking. Then it dawns on me: *they are assuming I am going to reconstruct.* One specific question is from a friend of mine who is also an RN. Perhaps, she has seen this so many times before, she just reasons I will be doing the same. I say, "Well, hopefully never. Actually, for me, I opted out of that." It is an awkward moment. "Oh! That's great!" she says. "My aunt made the same decision. She decided, at her age, why bother. She's been quite content ever since!" Find out later her aunt was almost seventy at the time.

This is what I've gathered reading a bit off the internet. Women who choose no reconstruction seem to fall into two general categories: (1) ultra-feminist types ("Burn the bra! Who needs these things! Plastic surgeons are sexist!") and (2) little-old-lady types ("What's the point? At my age, this old body is just falling apart anyway. No need to even keep up the pretense here.").

I have a hard time, honestly, because I fall into neither category. When I first had to pause and ponder, I could honestly not articulate why I decided against it; it was just a knee jerk, "not for me" type of gut reaction. Dr. Tuttle picked up on that immediately during our first office visit; I never even met with a plastic surgeon. But later on, having less anxiety, thinking it through, I believe there were really two reasons: (1) the end result and (2) avoiding unnecessary risk.

I have many women in my clinic panel who survived breast cancer and did go on to have reconstruction. I've been surprised, almost a bit taken aback, during the physical exam, when I lower the gown and I've temporarily forgotten about this particular aspect of their medical history. At times, I have found myself thinking, *That's a breast? Oh wait, I guess that's why they call it a breast "mound."* Because sometimes the resemblance to an actual breast—the shape, the feel, the look, the lack of a nipple—well, in some cases, takes a bit of a stretch of the imagination, honestly. And I know from a medical standpoint, this breast mound is going to be numb, no sensation, no intact erogenous zone. In my mind, it has no purpose other than filling out a silhouette in clothing. And now it seems I've come up with my perfect solution for that—the athletic bra with removable pads. In fact, I wish more women knew about that option. I see on the blogs some concern about wearing a silicone prosthesis inside a specialized bra that is heavy and uncomfortable, causing the skin to sweat excessively. For a woman who is an A or B cup, the athletic bra works amazingly well. It is soft and so comfortable to wear—even up against a healing incision. I will never need silicone—inside *or* outside my chest wall—and I think that's fantastic.

Then it seems some women indicate they pursue bilateral mastectomy to reduce the perceived cancer risk in the opposite breast—even though multiple studies enrolling hundreds of patients have shown this not to be the case. Other women state they want to make it easier to achieve symmetry with the plastic surgery approach. Well, to me, in these cases not only are you removing a perfectly healthy breast, risking surgical complications for no cancer benefit, but you are giving up the only functional side in terms of sensation, innervation, erogenous zone, and so on. This is the ultimate extension, a very unfortunate one in my opinion, of "the end result." While I know these decisions are entirely personal, with no one right answer, I just have to pause. I sincerely hope that women are completely informed as to what they are *actually getting* when they choose either option, because as far as an erogenous zone, well, it's kind of like donating a kidney for transplant: you really only need one for all practical purposes.

The other reason (unnecessary risk) was directly related to my training as a physician. Breast reconstruction involves multiple surgeries, many steps, each one carrying its own risks. I have seen too many complications over the years from something that was perceived to be a "minor" intervention. The bile leak after cholecystectomy performed to treat vague abdominal symptoms. The DVT and PE after foot surgery. I have even seen, just once, a perforation from a routine colonoscopy.

I even think back to complications that I have directly caused. I'm trying to place a central line, as an intern, in a patient in the ICU with very bad COPD and hyperinflated lungs, with no ultrasound guidance. Suddenly, we are drawing back air, and the resident and I look at each other with wide eyes. The patient sits up and says, "Oh, God," and becomes acutely short of breath. A pneumothorax. Fortunately, it's the middle of the afternoon; I pull off my gown and gloves and walk next door where the attending Dr. Craig Weinert is rounding and explain what just happened. He looks at me, sighs, and says very matter-of-factly, "Go get the chest tube tray." Minutes later, chest tube in, the patient's doing fine. He's sitting up and watching TV, and I am in the call room with my feet propped up on a chair from a near vasovagal episode.

Unfortunately, there is no procedure, no operation, no medication, no diagnostic test that is zero risk other than potentially a placebo. Doctors will know this, and likely be unable to separate that from their own medical decision making, regarding their own case management. On the other hand, I do recognize there are many women who may choose reconstruction because the psychological benefit outweighs the low risk of complications; an entirely valid approach. But as physicians, I think we tend to remember or recall more of the bad outcomes than good, making us potentially more risk averse.

This is probably why doctors also make terrible patients for certain things such as routine screening; they see both advantages and disadvantages of ordering more tests. Ironically, I once saw a forty-year-old female oncologist as a new patient, and we discussed screening mammography; she insisted on waiting until age fifty, and I thought at the time, *Well, if she is opting for that, so can I.* When we relocated to the new clinic building, we actually had problems one afternoon with internet access. Epic was down for a couple of hours, and I saw a female orthopedic surgeon for her routine physical. I asked her, "When was the last time you had a pap smear?" She said, "Oh, I am just not sure, maybe 3 years ago?" Since I couldn't check the chart, I went ahead and did it anyway. After internet access was restored, I entered the Health Care Maintenance tab and saw that *eight years* had elapsed since her last pap. *Typical MD*, I thought.

I look at my calendar; it's been six weeks since the operation. While it seems so long ago, it's still fairly recent. I try to think back, *When was the last time my appearance changed this drastically? Was it pregnancy? Was it dying my hair red in medical school?* Side note: I was playing Dr. Beverly Crusher from *Star Trek: The Next Generation* in a skit put on by the second-year medical students for the faculty. I accidentally used permanent hair dye to achieve this look when here I thought it was a temporary color. But then again, my friend Nick shaved his head to play Jean Luc Picard.

I also start listing in my mind what the alternatives could have been. If I could have had a lumpectomy and not a mastectomy, it might have been less noticeable, but I would have needed radiation treatment. If I had chosen reconstruction currently, I would be pumping saline into tissue expanders on a regular basis, which doesn't sound very fun to me at all. Then facing multiple follow-up surgical decisions: TRAM flap? Implant? And so on.

So first, give it more time, I tell myself. I'm going to have to draw on some inner reserves of some sort, those that have to do with appearance, self-image, body confidence, whatever we call it these days.

Consider the following from 1 Peter 3–4:

3   Your beauty should not come from outward adornment, such as elaborate hairstyles and the wearing of gold jewelry or fine clothes.
4   Rather, it should be that of your inner self, the unfading beauty of a gentle and quiet spirit, which is of great worth in God's sight.

I decide that for the time being, I will choose to focus on the inner self and not worry so much about the outward appearance. And I think about how much I'm enjoying the peace and quiet, the calm feeling, just being in the moment. I certainly don't need any more ups and downs. That will come later. After all, it's summer. Valleyfair is now open, and we live mere blocks from the State Fairgrounds. I can *choose* to go on those wild rides on my own free will, with each lasting less than three minutes in duration—perfect. That's enough excitement for me right now.

Chapter 29

TELEMEDICINE (PART II)

Not everybody trusts paintings,
but people believe photographs.
—Ansel Adams

Mid-June, the Internal Medicine Residency Program holds a dinner and program to honor the graduating residents. It became affectionately known as the Prom, many years ago because it is semiformal and everyone dresses up and puts on airs. It starts to become our mini version of the Oscars because after seeing each other continually in scrubs or in a boring long white coat over business attire, it is actually quite fun to see what other people are wearing. That's almost as important as who gets the award for Teacher of the Year or Best Diagnostician.

As I am getting ready for this evening, I am rummaging through my closet, and I realize that given my recent weight loss, many of my clothes just don't fit well anymore, including a few of the more formal dresses reserved for the Prom, the Oratorio Society Gala, or some awards dinner. One of my favorites is a black satin sheath with a sparkly jeweled neckline complete with black satin evening bag to match, but I bought it right after Lydia was born, probably the heaviest I had been in a while. It was for an awards dinner for Paul—he won the Residential Architects Vision and Excellence (RAVE) Award for Best Project under 800

Square Feet. I think this was my first big outing postpartum, and I was excited to get out of the house, Lydia being only a few weeks old at the time. So I had to run out and spend the money and buy this new dress even though I hadn't lost the baby weight yet. I really should get it taken in at some point, so I can wear it again.

This time, instead, I decide on a simple strappy Audrey Hepburn-esque cocktail dress; it's been in my wardrobe for a long time, and luckily, it still fits perfectly. But after zipping it up and looking in the bathroom mirror, I frown. I am wondering what is going on here; I can start to see some funny-looking contractures in my right arm. There are these band-like, raised, flesh-colored, ropy structures just under the skin in the axilla and also down in the antecubital fossa, extending across the inner elbow, actually quite visible to the naked eye. I wonder what on earth that could be. But I am in a hurry, late as usual, trying to get the kids fed dinner and me out the door before the program starts at 7:00 p.m. I drive to campus, park in the University Avenue Ramp, and make my way over to the reception room at TCF Stadium.

It is a very nice event. It's great to mingle with everyone there, including many faculty members that I normally don't get to see, from Regions and the VA. I also connect with several of the trainees, including two of our clinic residents, Eric and Mithun, whom I've worked with very closely over the past three years. Each of the twenty-eight graduates has selected a mentor to write something to send in a few comments about them to be read out loud at the ceremony; several ask me to do this, and I have no difficulty whatsoever composing glowing remarks regarding their incredible work ethic, dedication to patient care, and broad and deep knowledge base. One resident, Tyler, has obviously selected Dr. Charles Moldow; I can tell it is his writing as the piece is filled with self-deprecating humor: "It was really Tyler who taught the primary-care faculty and not the other way around." It is heartwarming for me to hear these comments being read out loud, not just to the benefit of the residents but to our faculty, the program directors, and our department chair. I so wished Charlie could have been there at the time.

But still, at the event, I keep looking down at my arm while I am listening to the graduates' names being read off and learning about their future plans. What the heck *is* that? I've been trying to engage in those home PT exercises; it helps a little, but now I am thinking about it, worrying a bit. Maybe I should have started the exercises sooner. I waited way too long, I bet. This is the sequela of babying that right arm and shoulder for the past month and a half, not wanting to aggravate any pain. I am doomed to a life of restricted mobility as well as this new and rather unattractive change in appearance. However, I'm still completely puzzled by it; I only know about lymphedema from my own clinical experience. This is different; it doesn't look the same. There is no swelling, and it appears instead as though there is a vine sprouting up from just above the incision, growing into the armpit, extending down the inner arm and sending out multiple shoots in different directions.

Of course, the graduation dinner is on a Saturday—why is it that everything always happens on a Saturday!—and I am trying to figure out what this is and what to do next. All the while I am wondering, questioning myself: Was it something I didn't do, such as range of motion exercises or *something I did do* to cause this to happen? If this is scar tissue, why did it seem to appear overnight, this far out from surgery? I think about heavy lifting while doing yard work, that tightening in my chest wall during my first run, other potential injuries. I wonder if I nicked myself shaving in the right armpit and somehow triggered inflammation. Could it be an odd presentation of a blood clot? Do I have a wound infection? Later when I look in the mirror, it doesn't appear that way, although there is one small spot that looks like a cross between a blister and a zit in the middle of the incision. It kind of hurts. I think it is because I am running a lot and the weather is warmer and I am getting sweaty underneath the nylon tank top. It has maybe caused a small area of chafing or perhaps a folliculitis, but I don't like the fact that it's smack dab in the middle of the incision. How can I get a wound infection over six weeks post-op? It's so tiny, though, I decide that can't possibly be the root of the problem.

On Sunday morning, I look again in the bathroom mirror, completely exposed chest. With the early morning light coming in through the window, I actually see another one of these flesh-colored "vines" extending straight down from the bottom edge of the incision, midline, down my trunk, ending just above the lower border of my right ribcage. Ugh! *What is this?* I go to my tablet, search PubMed and Google, but when I type in "contracture after mastectomy" what I get in return is a bunch of information regarding capsular contracture, which is a complication of reconstruction around the implant, or multiple studies related to post-op radiation. I keep thinking, *That ain't me. This is not me either.* I try different search terms, but I am getting nowhere fast. I give up and decide to contact somebody about this on Monday. And besides, Sunday morning there is church. I have to take Sam to a pool party that afternoon, and I need to finish planting annuals in the urns on the back patio. It's much, much later than I would normally be doing this, given everything going on. I will have to wait until Monday morning when everyone is back and contact the Breast Center with a question.

On Monday morning, first, I decide to send another staff message to Dr. Tuttle's nurse, Susan. I had reasoned this seems like something more surgical, possibly related to the operation, and that's where I would start. Although, again, I was totally confused about why new findings would appear six weeks out. I click into my own chart in Epic and compose a staff message, describing what I am seeing. I ask if she or Dr. Tuttle knows anything about this. At the same time, Charlie and I are still, as usual, e-mailing each other updates. I tell him, "I'm developing some sort of weird scar tissue or contracture or other complication, some ropy-looking thing in my right arm. Maybe I should contact the Breast Center?" He e-mails a response, first concerned that it could be a DVT (he's a retired hematologist, after all), then reminding me that Dr. Tuttle is in China all week.

Crap. Again, the timing of these things. Exquisite! It's a Monday morning, Monday being the only day I don't see scheduled patients in the office, so often I take advantage of that and work part of the day from home. I'm still working on my curriculum mapping in our online course management system known as BlackBag; I had planned on doing that from my home computer, then going in for afternoon meetings starting at 1:00 p.m. But I contemplate this new situation and consider what to do next.

I start to draw upon my recent past experiences and think about Charlie sending me electronically that photo of his post-op wound. I even think back to the Baltimore conference,

MedBiquitous, all about utilizing technology to further along medical education and patient care. What I really need is someone to just look at this and tell me what it is. There is actually a lot of medical literature around the therapeutic effect of "naming." If you can just tell someone what something *is,* give it a real-sounding medical diagnosis, a *name,* somehow that has a therapeutic effect in and of itself.

Consider this story: Very early in my career, I saw a middle-aged man, mid- to late forties, in my clinic for the symptom of chest pain. It was a second opinion of sorts; he brought a stack of medical records with him from all over the Twin Cities. I entered the room and shook his hand; I could tell, already, he was pretty anxious about this. "I just want answers. I need to find out what is going on." I asked him to describe his symptoms.

"I have been having chest pain, on and off, for six months now. I've been to several cardiologists. I even had an angiogram, which showed clean coronary arteries. They keep saying 'It's not this' or 'We've ruled out that,' but nobody seems to have a clue what could be actually causing the pain! I was told I should come to the U, that I need an expert opinion."

But back then, I was maybe two years out of residency and did not consider myself anywhere near expert. I swallowed hard. I thought, *Gee, I don't know anything more than the cardiologist you just saw for this exact same symptom! Help! And this patient seems well informed, obviously quite intelligent. He's extremely bright and even uses a lot of medical terminologies to describe both his symptoms and also the recent workup.* But I took a deep breath and asked him to hit pause, back up, and describe the pain in more detail.

"I'd say, the pain is somewhat variable, but it is usually sharp, and worse when I take in a deep breath." I asked him if it changed with position. "It does seem better if I sit up and lean forward." One of his many EKGs, I reviewed with interest. It had some very subtle, diffuse, upsloping ST elevations in multiple leads. That can indicate pericarditis, especially together with pain that is pleuritic and positional; but the rest of the EKGs were completely unremarkable. Still, I did a quick online literature search on the computer in the exam room, and I did find case reports and a small body of literature regarding pericarditis that is recurrent, thought to be possibly autoimmune in nature, maybe set off by a viral infection or some other inflammatory process that then comes and goes for years afterward.

After performing a detailed history and physical, I could tell he was upset. He was not happy that nobody could figure out what was going on. He described the dissatisfaction with multiple doctors, some who appeared to dismiss his symptoms. He also had a pretty high-stress job, working in IT, and admitted that not having an answer or even a suggestion as to what to do next was adding to his anxiety. I liked visiting with him; I felt the need to figure out some way to help him.

So I told him, "I think you may have chronic idiopathic recurrent pericarditis." I was totally going out on a limb here, to be honest, but it seemed at least as plausible as anything else. He said, "Really!" I explained to him my reasoning and that, while I had not seen this very often in my clinical practice (*not mentioning it's only been two years*), it was worth exploring. I also told him that the treatment seemed pretty simple and low risk in my estimation; it was NSAIDs for acute episodes, colchicine for prevention. He was extremely satisfied with this explanation and thought that I was a genius. He shook my hand upon leaving, and to this day (more than fourteen years later), he is still my patient. His visits to the ER or cardiology diminished rapidly after this, saving him time, unnecessary anxiety, and of course, health-care dollars. And all I did was give this a *name*, calling it a *syndrome*, and came up with a potential treatment plan.

Well, now, here I am in the same boat. I have no name for this; I need more information. And at the same time, I'm thinking about the wonders of telemedicine. If Charlie can e-mail a photo of his rear end to multiple providers, maybe I can do the same with my arm—at least it's not quite as intimidating as his anatomic region. And I can actually take a picture of this by myself without needing an assistant to run the camera. So I venture out on a limb, no pun intended, by sending yet another text message to Dr. Todd Tuttle.

"Heather here: quick question. I have these strange bands forming from my axilla down into the right arm, new over the past few days. Do you know what this is?"

He promptly replies: "I'm not sure. There is a thing called axillary web syndrome but usually associated with a lymph node dissection. Does it hurt?"

I text back: "It is tight, to be sure, but not really painful. Would a pic help?"

He replies: "Sure."

So then I go upstairs to my bathroom and try to figure out the best way to take a photo of this on my phone. First, I try it looking in the mirror, but that doesn't work as well. It's sort of blurry. Not able to see exactly what I am talking about, I take about a half dozen photos; I decide to focus on the right antecubital fossa with my arm extended completely. Ah, there it is. It appears as though there are guitar strings or fishing lines—whatever this may be just below the skin surface. But meanwhile, I am quickly googling "axillary web syndrome," and finally, yes, we have nailed it. The Google images are photos of exactly what I am seeing in the mirror, no doubt about it.

He replies: "If it persists, you might need to see a physical therapist. There is someone at the U who is interested in this condition."

I reply back: "Thank you! Never heard of this!" All the while, I am reading online that some of the risk factors are *younger age, low BMI.* Crazy! I certainly fit both of those. It seems pretty rare, though. There really is not a ton of literature out there, fewer than forty hits on PubMed. I also look this up in one of our go-to, quick online reference resources, Up to Date. You know you are really in trouble when Up to Date lists only a very brief paragraph that ends with "Further research is needed in this area."

But I am so thankful just to have the *name* of this condition. My earlier searches were completely useless; I was using the wrong terminology. I text back: "Thanks for the advice. Just knowing what the heck it is is very helpful! Have a good trip." I sit back, satisfied, enjoying this feeling, this moment of clarity.

I think back to my patient scenario mentioned above. Yes, naming seems to has a positive effect even if it changes absolutely nothing in terms of the treatment, the prognosis, and the outcomes—mostly because it gives you a way to find out more information. Although, at times, naming may have gone too far in medicine. It's really tempting in some ways as a physician to make up a diagnosis just to stop the endless barrage of laboratory testing, imaging, and referrals that accompany the unknown. I've had to say to some patients, "Many would say there is no such thing as chronic Lyme disease." Is that what I did possibly with my pericarditis patient? I think back to that old Seinfeld episode, where Elaine is trying to explain to her boss her father's medical condition. She tries to say with conviction and authority, "He is suffering from . . . oh, you know, neuritis. *Neuralgia.*" I wonder if that is how I sounded when I said *chronic idiopathic recurrent pericarditis.* At least I used four big words instead of one—a higher chance of success.

To this day, we will never know if I was right or wrong; certainly, we did not go back to the cath lab for a pericardial biopsy to figure it out. But at least I am still following him to monitor symptoms and to be sure that I did not miss something in my assessment; that's another huge strength of primary care. I don't pass people off; I hang on to them like a collector, amassing a veritable museum of pathology. Certain diagnoses, too, they just take time to sort out.

I recall my young male patient eventually diagnosed with systemic lupus; I usually think African-American females with this disease, and he's a big strapping Irishman complete with red hair and freckles. That might have been part of the problem, to begin with. Initially, he presented with a blood clot, then later low platelet counts, then finally, back pain and a urine specimen full of blood and protein. I had to string together these multiple episodes to come up with the correct unifying diagnosis and get him to a rheumatologist. Seeing patients back over time is often needed. "Tincture of time" is another saying in medicine—meaning, either the symptoms will resolve on their own, or something will happen to make the diagnosis more clear.

But if time also supposedly heals all wounds, well, I'm not sure how this applies to me and this new finding or what to do next. After reading more, it appears axillary web syndrome has been treated with physical therapy using specific massage techniques. I cringe when I read a relatively recent paper, May 2016, about a small case series of women having these bands injected by plastic surgeons with an enzyme called collagenase and percutaneous needle cord disruption with autologous fat grafting. Hmm, that sounds a little too invasive for me. I like the idea of PT much better. There are also descriptions of the bands spontaneously resolving on their own, sometimes in a matter of weeks to months. That would be great, in my opinion. Ignore the symptoms until they go away! I'm a pro at that! I've been doing it all my life—well, except for this one time, I guess.

I decide anyway that I'll just sit on this for now and think about it some more. Susan does reply to my initial staff message, giving me the name, phone number, and e-mail address of someone in the physical therapy program who has an interest in this condition. It's a fine start, and when I look up at my clock, it's not even 10:00 a.m. on that same Monday. Had I tried to phone the call center around 8:30 a.m., I am pretty sure I would have still been on hold by now. I am once again amazed by the power of technology and increasing the speed of getting answers. We simply must think about more ways to use this to integrate it into the everyday practice of medicine.

Chapter 30

THE DRIVING RANGE

They call it golf because all of the other
four letter words were taken.
—Raymond Floyd

T
he next day, I do get to speak with a physical therapist
very interested in this condition, *axillary web syndrome.*
She is a woman named Linda Koehler. She's very pleasant,
and even though by now I've read every article cited in PubMed
since the disorder was first described, I find the conversation
interesting and informative. She calls me on the phone and asks,
"Are you fairly thin? Active? Have you started exercising again?"
Her questions literally stopped me in my tracks as I am walking
and talking on my mobile. I think, *How does she know me so well?*

I tell her, "I ran twelve miles in the past three days."

She says, "There is a theory this happens in younger, thinner,
and physically active women because it is the injured lymph
system trying to reconstruct or regenerate itself."

And the physical activity may actually be causing some
of this, she says, stimulating in some way a much more robust
response. She tells me the axillary web has even been described
in elite athletes in the absence of surgery. She also asks me about
my limitation in terms of range of motion of that right arm. I
mention the difficulty in playing basketball with my kids, how
a right-handed layup is almost impossible. "Well, in my opinion,

that's really important. My son also plays basketball!" I tell her that I also play golf but I have been too chicken to find out what this has done to my swing.

That's true, actually; I have recently found myself more worried about golf than the pickup basketball game. Over the years, golf has become a big part of my life. It's always been one of those "date nights" for me and Paul, although less frequently than prior to having kids. It's so hard to find a babysitter. Still, Sam and Lydia are old enough to stay at home by themselves for a brief outing. We should be able to sneak out for a short round, maybe nine holes instead of eighteen, this coming season. Also, it's been great to play around with my female friends, such as Jodie or, in the past, JoAnn prior to her move. It's really nice to have someone along where we can both tee off from the same ladies' tee box." It's also a great excuse to get out and do something active while still talking, visiting, and catching up. It's our version of the coffee shop or the lunch deli or the happy hour, although we still do those things too.

Golf has also become a part of our regular vacation destinations. As it turns out, there are several family-friendly golf resorts. Some of the nicest are in Scottsdale, Arizona, where vacationers can drop off children in the "kid's camp" for supervised activities while parents play golf. Brilliant! I think, *Who was the sweet genius that came up with that idea?* In fact, both Jodie's family and my family took a vacation at the same resort in March of 2012. The two of us, plus our husbands, made up the golf foursome, and her three kids and my two kids had a great time together with the camp counsellors. They took them on treasure hunts, designed creative craft projects, supervised swim time at the pool, and even hosted a "digital" party where they made music videos and recorded movies to capture the memories. We all had such a great time. We had even talked about planning to do this again when, after our return, suddenly, without warning, Jodie's husband separated, moving out abruptly; they were divorced three years later. This was a shock, a terrible trauma to us all. Jodie and I are still very close, and we make efforts to get the kids together too, but it's much harder now with the complicated parenting schedule.

Still, my family of four has been back to that same resort since then and very much enjoyed it. So I am thinking, with this "web" thing going on, I really need to know what I can and cannot do. I leave work on a Thursday, a little after 5:00 p.m. It's a nice evening, warm but not too hot with a light breeze. I usually drive right by the University of Minnesota Les Bolstad Golf Course on my way home from work; along the north edge of Larpenteur Avenue sits the driving range. I have my clubs and two pairs of golf shoes in the back of my vehicle as always from March through November of any given year. Today, as I am passing by, I decide to heck with it; I make a left-hand-turn signal and pull into the parking lot.

I find an empty spot, park the rig, go around to the back cargo area, and pull out my golf bag. *Ooh, ouch*, even that hurts the right arm just a little bit. I place it on the ground; the kickstand snaps into place. I have to dig around and find an elastic hair band to pull my hair back in a ponytail. I kick off my heels, slip on the soft spike shoes, and pull the white mesh and leather glove onto the left hand. This is a routine I've done a thousand times before, but this time, I am actually feeling quite nervous. My heart rate is speeding up; my palms are sweaty. I look around; one thing about the university golf course, even the driving range—it is sure almost 100 percent men. Not a single feline to be seen among the canines. The course itself actually plays quite long and gives very little advantage off the tee to the women. On hole number 4, a very lengthy par 4, the ladies' tee is probably not even five yards in front of the men's. The other small thing I dislike about this course is that the driving range is not my favorite because it's all uphill. You can pick a target but then must realize that the elevation and a little bit of wind are probably going to subtract ten yards, which is a bit discouraging. But it's so convenient, right on my way home from work, that this is the range I frequent the most. And I still play the U course quite often. It's well maintained, and there are so many beautiful old growth trees that, in the fall with the changing of the leaves, it will make for a spectacular display of color.

This time, I am honestly just hoping I will be able to simply make contact with the ball without falling to the ground in agony. I slip my golf bag straps over both shoulders; that actually feels really good—the weight of the entire bag sort of stretching out my chest wall, relaxing the tension just a bit. I walk up to the counter and purchase a small bucket of balls, thirty in total. I hand the teenage lad my six dollars, grab the handle, and walk onto the range. I find the first open spot along the ropes and set up, dumping the bucket of balls onto the ground, bright yellow Titleist balls with the range markings.

I look at my clubs in the bag; should I start with a pitching wedge? An 8-iron? Now, I need quick answers here. I pull out the driver, a TaylorMade, slip off the head cover. I fish a long white tee out of the side pocket; I am *really* nervous now. The young guy next to me in the red polo, black pants, and white cap is just crushing it ball after ball with his Ping driver, I swear over three hundred yards, and it is intimidating me all the more.

So I do a few shoulder shrugs, grab the club like a handlebar, and try to stretch out just a bit. Then I bend over, tee up the ball, step back, and seek out a target. There's a bright-red flag slightly to the left of center, and when I check the yardage board, it says 162. Perfect! Remember, I will have to subtract ten yards to mimic normal, and if I can drive the ball straight 150, I'm happy. On rare occasion, if I actually approach 175 yards, I will break into a dance. It's the slice that always gets me, taking off potential distance and usually landing near the right side of the fairway.

My usual pre-shot routine includes a practice swing, which doesn't feel too bad. There is no pain, no limitation that I can tell; and considering the mechanics of a golf swing, even for a right-handed golfer, it is truly the left arm that is most important. It must always take the lead. The right arm gets out of the way; it should just be along for the ride. The left arm needs to pull the club through, closing the clubface at the point of contact with the ball. If the right arm is too active, overzealous, that is the nature of a slice or a block where the clubface is open and every shot lands to the right. It's actually quite difficult for a right-hand-dominant person to do this, which is why players spend years trying to get the slice out of their swing, and it's why golf is honestly just a messed-up game, to begin with. Incredibly challenging, to say the least.

Well, *here we go*, deep breath. I begin the backswing, pause at the top, rotate my torso, give it all I've got, and *ping*. The ball sails through the air, perfect arc, slight fade, lands just to the near right of the red 162-yard flag and rolls well beyond. *What the—?* That was much, much better than I ever thought possible even before the surgery. I conclude this must be a fluke. I hit two more in rapid succession, but they land almost exactly in the same place, a little farther even. Same roll forward until I see three of my bright-yellow balls lined up within a foot of each other beyond the red flag in a perfect row, like an ellipsis.

Huh, unbelievable. I slip the head cover back on the driver and trade it for my 3-wood, then my 5-wood, then 7-iron. I hit every single club in my bag, each one the same distance or better than the previous. And a bit of a draw instead of a slice! I can hardly believe it; I am very relieved, so grateful. And as I look around me, taking in the entire scene, I realize nobody else on this driving range could possibly appreciate what this means to me or how big of a deal this is. Then all at once, I find I have only five balls left on the ground. I switch back to the driver just for fun and power through those last few range balls. *Ah the sound of it.* I feel very satisfied.

But I then realize, oops, I forgot to call home and tell them I would be a bit late. I quickly finish up. I rush to the car, throw everything in the back, change shoes, and pull out my wallet and mobile from my golf bag and see a text. I get in and reply, "On my way," and speed just a bit on the drive back to our house.

I walk through the front door with a big grin on my face and announce, "Guess what I just did!" Sam and Lydia are sitting on the couch, looking very annoyed. I glance at the clock, and it's 6:35 p.m. I realize they are just hungry for dinner. Suddenly I feel terrible; I am turning into an awful, selfish, neglectful mother. At times, it is like I am in my own little world. But I also have been thinking about this recently, realizing, hoping (rationalizing?) that in clearing some of these hurdles, such as the first run, the first golf swing, and so on, it will eventually cease to be an issue. It will restore me back to the point where I can turn fully toward *them* and focus once again on taking care of my family. It's similar to the instructions they give you on the airplane: in the event of loss of cabin pressure, secure your own mask before assisting others. Although things are going well for me on so many levels, I have to admit, I am still very much in the process of securing my own mask.

Paul comes in from outside in the backyard, and I tell him excitedly about my amazing success on the driving range. He states matter-of-factly, "Well, of course. This is because your right arm is restricted." Ever the architect, he goes on to talk about the architecture of the swing. He describes how there is a drill taught by the golf pros where they place a towel under the right arm, and you are supposed to follow through on the entire swing without letting the towel drop, to keep that right arm quiet, up close against the body, and thereby preventing a slice. He even mentions that this was one of the weak spots in Jack Nicklaus's swing. He has a tendency to "wing" his right arm, which somehow works for him but with potentially disastrous results for an amateur. I just have to indulge in a good laugh honestly, and I say, "Blessings in disguise this axillary web syndrome, I guess!"

The next day, a Friday, is my full day marathon clinic, as usual. I also happen to see, in Epic, that Dr. Anne Blaes has clinic that same morning, two floors below me. After I did my lit search, I found out that she is a coauthor on a paper regarding this condition. Amazing! Yet another reason I am so glad she is my oncologist. I wonder if I should e-mail her or send her a staff message or just show up. Unlike Dr. Tuttle, she's currently located on *this* continent, so I decide to stop by in person.

At around 11:00 a.m., I am in between patients, and I use our high-tech locator badge system to see that Dr. Blaes is in the 2E collaboration zone. I bolt down the two flights of stairs and walk back there to find where she is at. She is sitting at a computer, dictating a note. Dictation? I think. Wow, am I the only physician who types my own notes? What a sucker I have been all these years! But as soon as she sees me, she hits pause and looks up to say hello with a big smile. I ask, "Can I have a minute of your time?" We go to find an empty exam room. This feels like the umpteenth time I have simply arrived in clinic unannounced and accosted one of my physicians. I sincerely hope I am not wearing out my welcome. I pray that they will still take care of me despite multiple text messages or me barging in. Dr. Tuttle probably dreads seeing my number pop up on his phone. I am thinking, I should really send more cards or a box of chocolates, something to let them know how much I appreciate all this. I wonder if they like pickled beets or homemade salsa.

I say, "I just have to show you something." I extend my arm and point out the "web" and mention this is new over the past few days, and she says, "Oh, wow." I tell her about the text to Dr. Tuttle and how we figured out it was axillary web syndrome. She does a brief exam, feeling the cords in the antecubital fossae as well as the axilla. "This is pretty dramatic. I don't usually see visible bands this far down into the forearm." That makes me feel so much better; I was freaking out a bit honestly over the past week before I knew what this was. But the fact that even *she* is impressed means I wasn't overreacting to the situation. It's such a fine line honestly, knowing what to do, when to call, how to even *respond* or *react* regarding a potential complication. I think back to Gay Moldow's e-mails; she is very much spot-on.

But then I do tell Anne I have already discussed over the phone the situation with our resident expert Linda Koehler. I mention I've been trying some home exercise regimens, but she now recommends a formal physical therapy assessment. "You really need to see someone in person."

"Great, no problem," I tell her. "I will schedule that right away."

She goes to the computer, puts in the referral, and gives me the phone number on a sticky note to call for the appointment. Lastly, trying to boost her mood, I tell her about my adventure to the driving range first time since surgery. Not knowing if she plays golf or not, I tell her, "I think these webs are actually helping my golf game by restricting my right arm just enough to eliminate my slice." She is truly laughing out loud now as I stand up and demonstrate with a phantom swing how it keeps my right arm close to the body and I had such amazing success at the driving range last night. She seems entirely amused. "You and your e-mail updates have been cracking me up and providing much-needed entertainment."

I reply, "That's my job. Just trying to bring some humor and laughter into this place." It's true; it's become almost a calling.

I leave the 2E collaboration zone and walk back up the stairs to finish my morning clinic session. I am now feeling so much better about this entire situation. Over the past five days, from finding out *what this is* from Dr. Tuttle to chatting on the phone with Linda, to having Dr. Blaes see me in person—they all have brought me from that panicky place of the unknown to having a plan going forward. It seems small, probably to them, but it's a big deal to me. Although as I am standing at my workstation in the 4B collaboration zone, I am once again lost in thought, aimlessly going through the motions of my golf swing. I'm thinking, Huh, if I do get physical therapy and completely correct this problem, I could potentially go right back to my slice. That's sort of depressing, I must admit. Maybe this is truly the time to seek professional help *on all levels*. The University of Minnesota Les Bolstad Course hosts both private and group golf lessons at my very same driving range with two PGA pros. I look up the information online and think, *After the Fourth of July, this just might be some time well spent.*

Chapter 31

TAMOXIFEN

I need a remedy, for what is ailing me, you see.
If I had a remedy, I'd take enough to please me.
—Black Crowes

The question still remains about when to start tamoxifen. In my opinion, the best answer is never, but I realize that's probably not a good choice. I have a pale-blue bottle, a thirty-tablet supply, tamoxifen citrate (20 mg), sitting on the counter in my bathroom for weeks. I keep looking at it with some hesitation. I had even asked Dr. Blaes, given my Oncotype assay result, "What is my *absolute* risk reduction with this drug?" In other words, what would happen if I didn't take it? (But notice, I didn't use those words.) "Your recurrence rate in that situation would be 10 percent, which is double the number of 5 percent, or the recurrence rate *with* tamoxifen." She gave me a slight look at the time, then said, "Everyone in this field would say you should be on tamoxifen." I felt a bit like a scolded child. *She's onto me.* But when I think about those numbers, I do know some women, friends of the family, and also my neighbor who refused to take tamoxifen but instead turned to herbal remedies or following a low-estrogen diet or a host of alternative approaches.

In fact, I've actually been handed a package of bona fide Chinese medicinal herbs from a friend of mine who recently joined our moms' group. She's from China and a pharmacist by training, but now she is a stay-at-home mom of two young girls. Her husband is an engineer at a local medical device company. In the past year, she had an abnormal mammogram, and fortunately, the biopsy came back negative. Before she knew this, however, she contacted her family back in China, and they sent her an entire shipment, several crates of a Chinese herbal remedy that supposedly cures breast cancer. Each one week of daily dosing comes wrapped in an orange cellophane wrapper; it is covered, of course, in Chinese writing. At a visit to her house, Jin-Fang offers to give some to me and to translate the ingredients and instructions.

I take one package home as a souvenir of sorts and place it on my countertop, next to the pale-blue tamoxifen bottle. "*Xiao Jin Wan*," it says across the top; I go to Google Translate and type it in, and I hear the correct pronunciation. However, typing into Google Search routes me directly to PubMed. First article: "Xiao Jin Wan, a traditional Chinese herbal formula, inhibits proliferation via arresting cell cycle progression at the G2/M phase and promoting apoptosis via activating the mitochondrial-dependent pathway in U-2OS human osteosarcoma cells." How interesting. I am impressed by the preliminary research results, but question if they apply to *in vivo* use. Now, out of curiosity, I even go so far as to open the orange package. There are these very strange-looking white round balls with an orange dot on the top. They look like fishing bobbers to me. Peering more closely, I think I can see something inside. I try to cut one open with scissors, but it doesn't work. Do patients swallow these whole? They are at least an inch in diameter. Maybe they dissolve in hot water? Eventually, I place the package in my purse for the next time we are dining out at our local Chinese restaurant, our regular night, every Tuesday, corner booth. I show the package to our waitress and ask her how one might go about taking these. She shows me the "seam" on the side of this white ball where you place a knife or a fingernail and pop it open; inside there are two dark-green tablets wrapped in plastic. I find myself wondering how this would compare to taking Tamoxifen. Although, I am aware of a lack of studies proving benefit from Chinese herbal medicine in terms of breast cancer outcomes.

I then start to wonder why, in adult medicine, we don't use weight-based dosing more often as we do in pediatrics. I find it interesting that we equate the same 20 mg dose in an adult female who weighs 110 pounds to potentially another patient who weighs 220; that's fully two of me. Would that not have some effect on the pharmacokinetics, the pharmacodynamics? Or maybe not. I have a PharmD colleague of mine, Keri, that I recently let in on my diagnosis. Maybe I will ask her for an opinion if I can try taking 10 mg instead. Or I could always e-mail Dr. Blaes.

Thinking about my half-dose strategy, though, I realize I'm just still fearful of the potential side effects. That is why I had wanted to wait until after my one week of inpatient attending to start taking it. I was imagining being on rounds with the team, coming up with plans for each patient, and feeling a wave of a hot flash come over me. Or, considering one of the side effects is fatigue; being on pager seven days in a row, I may get called in the middle of the night if one of our patients is crashing, which is tiring enough. Once I am back to a more predictable schedule of outpatient clinic, it seems more reasonable. And I had gotten permission earlier from Dr. Blaes. She was okay with this approach. I realize when you are discussing the benefits of taking a drug for the next five to ten years, a few weeks' delay is probably not going to make much difference.

So finally, end of June, I begin taking tamoxifen. I did end up starting with a half tablet at bedtime, then increased it to a whole tablet. And as far as monitoring for side effects, I think, *Well, it's going to be awfully difficult to tell what is what here. For some reason, I haven't been able to sleep past 5:00 a.m. since my diagnosis, end of March. Is that causing some mild fatigue? Gee, I have newly radically altered anatomy in an area that is somewhat important for intimacy. Could that be contributing to low libido?* I start to realize that almost everything reported in the way of side effects is nonspecific and could be completely and totally unrelated. The only one I can say with absolute confidence from my own experience is an ACE inhibitor inducing a cough.

But at the start, I am not experiencing any *major* hot flashes, just minor ones. After two weeks, I observe that I am just feeling much warmer than usual, constantly rather than in "flashes." I find myself wanting to wear sleeveless dresses and tank tops. I'm spontaneously shedding my white coat in clinic and repeatedly checking the thermostat at my house. Still, I think, well, maybe that's good. It means the drug is actually doing something. Sort of like my post-MI patients who are on both aspirin and clopidogrel. I don't mind if they report a minor nosebleed now and then.

After three or four weeks, I realize, gee, this drug must have a long half-life or just take some time to see the estrogen effect. Because now I'm rolling in the deep, really feeling it—not just warm all the time but coupled with more intense flashes two to three times a day. These hot flashes are very strange, not what I would have expected. They always start in my "core," usually the lower abdomen or pelvic area or even upper thighs. I will think, *Oh boy, here comes another one.* It's a searing sensation. The burning intensifies, then generalizes, usually concluding with my face turning red as a beet. Once in a while, they wake me up at night. I am wearing the lightest summer nightgown, a camisole with thin straps, with an oscillating fan blowing over me; but still, I wake up and kick off all the covers but to no avail. I am wondering to myself, *How long will this go on? It is entirely possible that these symptoms will lessen over time, right?*

Also, once again, I am puzzled by my weight. Every website, every internet blog, every patient information handout talks about *weight gain* on tamoxifen. I, however, have lost weight, even the few pounds I regained after surgery. Now I am down another five pounds down on top of the initial ten-pound loss, and this is despite eating normally. My appetite is definitely back; I am eating with abandon. Yes, I am back to running but no more than prior to this diagnosis. I consult once again my usual quick source, Up to Date, and read LexiComp drug information regarding tamoxifen. It says weight loss occurs in 26 percent of patients; weight gain, 9 percent. I might tend to believe up to date more than internet blogs. Or, the phase one trials that compared tamoxifen to placebo, and showed no difference in weight.

Now, again, most women would think weight loss was spectacular. Unfortunately, some of my loss of weight is also occurring—how should I say this—in *all the wrong places.* I lose the right breast to surgery, and then the left one simply melts away on tamoxifen. *Sheesh!* I read further online that tamoxifen has an off-label use for treating male gynecomastia. This makes perfect sense to me. I'm experiencing it first-hand and also consider the fact that we are blocking the effects of estrogen on breast tissue. I would think it could definitely cause some regression, so to speak; "shrinkage" to borrow that Seinfeld term. I try my best not to get upset by this; after all, this could have been the summer of chemo—Docetaxel and Cytoxan!—instead of just tamoxifen. But I have to admit, there are days when I pause and consider calling Dr. Umar Choudry. I am trying to imagine his response: "You come see me *now*?" This is exactly how I feel when I have a diabetic patient of mine present with a wound on the foot that has been smoldering for weeks.

But at the very least, I can say that I am honestly approaching perfect symmetry. This is the goal of every plastic surgeon after all. Thankfully, I don't seem to be experiencing any of the so-called brain fog, which was frankly my worst fear. And reading a bit further, I am actually encouraged by the beneficial effects of tamoxifen on bone density. Not only do I have a low BMI as a risk factor for osteoporosis, but Dr. Blaes checked my vitamin D level, and it was in the tank, quite low. I start taking a weekly capsule, 50,000 IU of vitamin D, then switch to a daily dose. This, along with tamoxifen, along with the candesartan, I am starting to feel like an old woman here needing all these pills! I keep getting calls from Walgreens at different times of the month, saying, "You need to come in and get your thirty-day refill." What a pain!

Through all of this, I can't help but whine just a bit to Paul. "Can't you adjust the thermostat upstairs? I am feeling warm and uncomfortable all the time, especially at night." I complain about my weight loss, which at this point has almost necessitated purchasing an entirely new wardrobe, which *sounds* great, but who has the time to shop? "I can't use online shopping. I need to try everything on. I have no idea what size I am. And I'm not sure I want to spend tons of money if I gain the weight right back." I decide I'll just have to buy a few more belts and eat more or simply wait a few months. There's nothing like a Minnesota winter to put a damper on running; that in combination with food around the holidays will certainly pack on some pounds.

Paul notices when I am constantly fiddling with the climate control in our car or the AC in our master suite; he's also expressed concern about my weight, saying I'm too thin. At one point, he suggests, "Maybe you should just stop taking it." While I was at times just complaining to garner a bit of sympathy, I must confess I had been considering that too. But on the other hand, even I, as a medication nihilist, think I should stay on tamoxifen for the long haul. I need to give it my very best effort. And one Sunday morning, in church, we have this point driven home for both of us in a moment of perhaps divine intervention.

My family of four is sitting in the back row as always; it's a few minutes before the start of the 11:00 a.m. service. Soft music is playing as people are filing in. Paul and I are sitting in the very last pew with Sam and Lydia seated in between us; we are both scanning the bulletin. There is a section at the end of page 2 for prayer requests, and in it, someone has submitted the following: "Please pray for my friend Brenda. She was diagnosed with breast cancer three years ago and had surgery and was doing great. Now, the cancer is back, and it's in her liver and her bones." Paul is reading through this, then leans over to look at me and points to the prayer request. I look back at him and just slowly nod.

He says, "This isn't the same type of breast cancer you have, is it?"

Oh yes, indeed, the very same one. But instead, I say, "Well, it's a later stage. It's a more aggressive form."

"But how can you get breast cancer in the liver or in the bones?"

Hmm. Maybe I should have brought you along to those oncology appointments. This is metastatic disease. Instead, I say, "Once breast cancer spreads, it can go anywhere. Liver and bone are pretty common."

And finally, the real kicker: "This couldn't happen to you, could it?"

It sure as hell could! I could be dead in five years! I then swallow hard, thinking, *Censor that, especially "hell." I'm sitting in church.* Instead, I pause, take a deep breath, and say, "Well, that's why I take tamoxifen." And that is the honest truth. Despite feeling as though I want to crawl out of my own skin from the hot flashes or losing weight or having other potential side effects and other complications down the road, I've just got to keep taking it to hopefully prevent this awful thing, a recurrence or metastasis, from ever happening.

But then I also say out loud to Paul, "There are no guarantees in life, and every day is a gift from God." Sam and Lydia are reading the children's bulletin; one is working on a crossword, and the other a word search. They glance up at us, wondering what we are talking about. Now, the piano playing stops. The musicians are taking the stage for the worship music, and our Pastor Todd Olson is approaching the pulpit. He asks us all to bow our heads in prayer. I can't help but immediately think, *Lord, help me stay on this miserable tamoxifen as long as it takes. Whatever side effects may come, give me the strength to endure it so I can be there for my family.*

I glance over at the three of them, Sam, Lydia, and Paul, sitting quietly in the pew, heads down. They are the real reason; they are my motivation for doing all of this. Because if I do ultimately succumb to breast cancer, it's not me who will suffer; I'll be in a better place, but certainly, at least for some time, they will not.

And that's why I continue to take tamoxifen.

Chapter 32

PHYSICAL THERAPY

The doctor of the future will prescribe no medicine but
will involve the patient in the proper use of food,
fresh air, and exercise.
—Thomas Edison

The other treatment option I need ASAP is exercise—more specifically physical therapy for this right arm to address the axillary web syndrome. I notice that while the golf swing anti-slice mechanism is great, pretty much *everything else* is not. Reaching up to place something on a high shelf, leaning over to grab my purse from the passenger seat in the car, washing my hair in the shower—these things are really difficult. That's when the tightness is quite noticeable. It's very restrictive, these crazy cords. When I took in the mirror with tangential lighting and stretch out my arm just so at the inner elbow, they honestly make my arm look like a six-string guitar. *I guess I am now finally fulfilling anatomically what they all say—that I am too high strung.* I am also trying to think of possible home remedies for the situation. There is an urban legend about how to manage a ganglion cyst in the wrist area. Slam the family Bible on it, and it will regress. I wonder if the same could be true for these bands. What if I use a closet door or something to really crank on it, fully engage the arm in hyperextension, and see what happens? Then once while getting dressed, this actually occurs on its own. I am pulling a T-shirt over my head when I feel a *snap, pting,* and a zinging sensation from my armpit all the way down to my wrist. Then a sudden slight loosening of the tension; it felt like the big Northern Pike that had just snapped the fishing line and got away. That was honestly one of the strangest physical sensations I have ever experienced in my entire life.

My first physical therapy visit is smack dab in the middle of the week of inpatient attending. I inform my team, apologizing since we are on call, "I've got a PT appointment this afternoon. I can still be available by pager. I should only be gone for about an hour." They are fine with it, and I also let the triage doc know as a backup since I will be physically located in a different building across the river. I ride the shuttle to the West Bank campus, also known as Riverside. I make my way over to the lymphedema treatment center and check in.

I get to meet a very nice woman named Carol. She's a tall, curvy, middle-aged lady with shoulder-length wavy brown hair who begins by taking several measurements in both arms, including circumference, grip strength, and range of motion. As I take off my top and bare my arm, she says, "Oh, wow, this is impressive." It's similar to Dr. Blaes's comment upon viewing for the first time. I begin to think, *I should take some more pictures of this at home for posterity's sake.* I have a post-op snapshot of me on my phone in the Bair Hugger about thirty minutes after waking up from anesthesia; this could be next in the photo album. How fun! I'll create a scrapbook later on!

She then goes on to teach me some stretching exercises and proceeds to do some sort of massage to the entire arm area, focusing on the cords; this is manual lymphatic drainage presumably to apply compression and start to move them in the right direction. It's not painful. It actually feels kind of good, and for a few minutes, I feel as though I am almost going to fall asleep. These early mornings, late nights are catching up with me. I also wonder, *How about a hot stone massage? Mani, pedi? Let's make this a spa day, one that I can even get excused from work, and have it covered by insurance.* After this, she takes some measurements again and finds that my range of motion has already increased even after just these simple interventions.

After some final assessments, she tells me to get dressed and gives me a packet of home instructions, more exercises to do on my own. She also mentions, "You should be wearing a compression sleeve whenever possible and especially for high-risk situations, such as airplane travel." She hands me a booklet, advertising these colorful arm sleeves called Lymphedivas. Inwardly, I think, *Thank you, Carol, but no way am I wearing one of those.* It's summer! I am sporting tank tops and sundresses! Talk about advertising to the entire world the fact that you have breast cancer and just had surgery. Not to mention, it would be hot and uncomfortable on a ninety-degree day, I presume. I just smile and nod and tuck the Lymphedivas pamphlet into the blue folder. After the visit, I think, *Wait, I already did fly to Baltimore and back, with no issues. The arm itself is not swollen to me at all, and it's not clear from the literature if axillary web syndrome is a risk factor for developing chronic lymphedema.* So I decide, I'm just going to skip that recommendation for now.

One week later, I come back to the same physical therapy location; but this time, I meet a petite, blond, athletic-looking woman named Lisa. She reviews Carol's notes and asks me, "How are the home exercises going?" I stare back blankly and then say, "Just great!" I think I maybe did this once in seven days honestly. I spent all week, including Saturday and Sunday, rounding and trying to prevent two of the patients from actively dying on us; they were in and out of "slow codes" as we call them, or critical care time in the billing world, where you feel as though you just can't leave the bedside until things get stabilized. But the problem with PT is, you actually have to do your homework to see the benefits. I start to think, *I am the worst patient in the world. I blew off the suggestion of the sleeve, I haven't done squat in terms of home exercises, and at this point, I haven't even started tamoxifen yet. For shame.*

But well, I am here right now, so even though I tell this little white lie, I do mention to Lisa about the improvement in range of motion and that I'm willing to try new and different exercises as she sees fit. She gets right down to business; she asks me to take off my shirt, and once again, I have yet another health-care provider marvel at the cords. I am starting to feel a bit like a circus freak. *Step right up and see the woman with the weird wide web.* She repeats some measurements, mostly arm circumference and range of motion again, but also pinches my skin in several areas to see if I have any swelling on the arms or the trunk or the upper back. It reminds me of when my junior high gym teacher used fat calipers to tell us about our body fat composition and shame us into doing more pushups.

Next, she has me lie down on the table and starts to massage my right arm, *but* unlike the previous visit, she's got a slightly more rigorous approach to this entire thing. She's really cranking on me, stretching out the arm, at one point leaning with most of her weight while I have the arm up above my head, fully extended back on a pillow. And as opposed to falling asleep, I have to admit, this time around, I am instead gritting my teeth for almost the entirety of the visit. At one point, she is massaging deeply and firmly into the area immediately above the incision and into the right axilla, which has two large ropy cords. It is triggering some very visceral reactions. It's slightly painful and uncomfortable, and it is actually causing me to experience waves of nausea. My mouth is salivating! I think, *What if I have to sit up and lean over and vomit on the floor?* This would not make for the best outcome for this encounter.

It's a few more minutes of enduring these odd and uncomfortable sensations, and finally, she lets up a bit. Instead, she has me stand up and demonstrate how I'll do some of these home exercises, such as the wall walking, the snow angel, and so on. However, upon measuring the range of motion again, we have found a huge benefit, even greater than before. The abduction of the right arm went from about 95 degrees to almost 130 degrees! I say, "I feel much more loose and limber now." I'm really motivated to do better for next time. I confirm that I have two more PT sessions scheduled; I leave with several additional instruction sheets.

Over the next two weeks, I am actually pretty good about doing these home exercises, at least once a day, sometimes two or three times a day. I am also fairly insistent in the clinic 4B collaboration zone, that I get first dibs on one of the four standing workstations out of the twelve in that area. I notice that if I am sitting too long at a computer desk, it just makes everything worse. I can't help but lean forward and hunch over the screen, and it contributes to the overall tightness. And these particular sit to stand workstations are all, very handily, next to an opposing wall;

so then as I am reviewing charts in Epic, I find myself "walking the wall" with my right arm as often at work as I do at home. At one point, my colleague Dave Macomber is sitting next to me on my left, staring at this motion, and asks, "What on earth are you doing?"

I give him a vague response: "My right arm needs physical therapy."

He says, "Oh, I thought we were all just making you crawl the walls out of some serious anxiety disorder or something."

I just laugh and tell him, "No, I go running for that."

The third weekly PT session, I meet Meghan. She's got curly chin-length golden-brown hair, tanned skin, and a petite but athletic physique. She greets me, and I tell her, "I think this is getting much better—not just the range of motion, but the cording seems to be regressing! The one on my trunk is gone. The axillary bands are much less prominent. Just those stubborn forearm bands remain."

She begins by performing her own measurements. "I agree, these numbers show improvement too." She wants me to demonstrate my home exercises; I enthusiastically jump up and lean against the wall, performing the snow angel, like an eager ballerina performing for the ballet maestro. After we do some stretching and massage therapy, she says, "I'd like to perform *cupping* on the bands in the antecubital fossa."

"Really?" I ask. "What on earth is that?"

Meghan replies, "It's an ancient Chinese technique which helps loosen up and release scar tissue, and it may do the same with the cording."

I say, "Okay, sure, let's try it. I've got China on the brain lately, that is for certain."

She gets out this vacuum-type device with Chinese characters on the side; she shows me how it works. It has a glass tube attached that applies a controlled level of suction to soft tissue. Next, she starts working on the bands in the elbow area. It gives me a tugging, gentle pulling sensation that I can feel all the way up into my healing incision. I then remember, I still have the Chinese medicinal herbs that supposedly cure breast cancer sitting in my purse, which is on a chair next to me. I decide to share with her that story. We both have a laugh, and after chatting for some time, she says, "I am a breast cancer survivor myself, eight years out." I congratulate her and think, *See, I'm not the only health-care provider who opens up to a few select patients.* After the cupping is completed, she sends me out with some more home instructions, this time for weight training. I will go home and find my ten-pound weights tucked in a storage closet upstairs, dig them out, and start biceps curls, chest presses, and triceps extensions.

My fourth and final visit, I get to see Carol again. That's a good thing; the therapist who evaluated me at the very first visit can now see what great progress has been made. She again examines the arm: "Wow, the cording is much less." She takes down the standard measurements, the grip strength, and the range of motion. She repeats the assessments for pain and disability, which have gone from a 3/10 and a 30/100 to zero. I have one last round of manual lymphatic drainage—which again feels akin to a spa massage—and one more round of "cupping" for those stubborn forearm bands. Only this time, she uses a different device—not the ancient Chinese vacuum but instead an emergency snakebite kit. How interesting! Instead of removing poisonous venom from a snakebite, it's instead lifting up on the cording as I feel a gentle pulling sensation. It's not quite as dramatic as the Chinese device, but afterward, it seems that everything is a bit looser. Carol then congratulates me and says, "You are officially discharged from PT. Our goals have been met. Continue the home exercises!"

So all in all, given what could have potentially happened at each of these steps along the way—the early detection of the cancer, tamoxifen instead of chemo, axillary web syndrome, which is rapidly improving—I realize I've been blessed. I am sitting at the Underground Music Cafe one Friday evening, listening to jazz, when I look down and see that even those funny-looking cords at the elbow are finally regressing. I can barely see them now unless I put traction on the skin and hold up my arm against tangential lighting. And more importantly, my right arm has been restored to completely normal range of motion; it's great to be able to reach up to the high shelves in my kitchen cupboards without calling for assistance. I'm even enjoying some new upper-body definition from the weight training, something I haven't done in years.

I did make use of my home digital camera, and early on, I had my family take some pictures of my arm when the cording was fairly prominent. Sam kept asking, "Mom, what *is* that? Eew!" I said, "Never mind, just snap a few more! Make sure the flash is on!" Paul came into the room and took some additional shots after seeing what Sam had done.

I look at those photos, and I think, *Hey, that's much more dramatic than what I saw on PubMed or Google Images.* I have a thought pop into my head. *Maybe I should write myself up as a case report?* Now that is truly poetic justice, to get an academic publication out of this for the CV. Wow! Later, Charlie and I share a big laugh about that over coffee one Tuesday morning. He thinks I should go for it and even suggests a few journals to target for submission.

At the time, I thought to myself, *Is it possible to be having "fun" with one's own cancer diagnosis?* Between writing a case report and a book about my experiences and forming strong bonds with other people over it, there are admittedly times when I honestly feel that way. It's been . . . *fun?* A *good* thing? If someone would have told me this on March 31 after the first appointment with the radiologist, I would have thought they were *insane.* Considering all this, I am glad I hung in there through the early weeks. I am grateful for everyone's support during that time because now, as I am able to reflect back, I can start to see the silver lining in this cloud, even ways to make lemonade out of lemons.

> Consider it all joy, my brethren,
> when you encounter various trials,
> knowing that the testing of your
> faith produces endurance.
> —James 1:2–3 (NASB)

I feel as though I am nearing a turning point where I *can* consider it all joy.

Chapter 33

BACK TO ORATORIO

Music is a moral law. It gives soul to the universe,
wings to the mind, flight to the imagination, and
charm and gaiety to life.
—Plato

Choral music is big in Minnesota. We are famous for the Saint Olaf Choir, established in 1912, as the premiere college choir with a national reputation, setting the standard for choral music excellence. And that's just in the little town of Northfield, Minnesota, with a population of twenty thousand. It is set among the farm fields with the motto: "Cows, College, and Contentment." In the Twin Cities, there are also many fine choral ensembles to be found, including VocalEssence, Cantus, and the Minnesota Chorale. I've been a part of the Oratorio Society of Minnesota since 1996—I just realized very recently that's twenty years. Twenty! Almost embarrassingly, I have been committed to this community choir longer than any other single endeavor in my life, including marriage, family, and career. I did sit out a few performances here and there, such as while on maternity leave or when I had to recertify, studying for and taking (again, lucky me!) the Internal Medicine Boards in 2012, but I always came back.

And again, in January of 2016, I sat out once more, thinking, *I need to get my Monday nights back temporarily. Rehearsal is every Monday, 7:00–10:00 p.m.* The main reason: Sam is now on the basketball team, and all of his games are on a Monday. And recently, Sam's trumpet skills got him recruited to the jazz band—a big deal, a great honor, but now he's committed to a very early Tuesday morning rehearsal—meaning, a late Monday isn't good for either of us. In fact, I pondered if I should ever come back to choir, given that things feel so much busier with two kids who are now involved in a bunch of activities and also have way more of a social life than me at this point. The invites keep coming in—birthday parties, after-school get-togethers, pool parties, sleepovers, bonfires.

In retrospect, knowing what I know now, the two performances in early April would have been a disaster; I was still completely panicked by the new diagnosis of breast cancer. And the concert? It was choral music set to a silent film *Joan of Arc*—all about death, dying, a bit grim and depressing. Just what I would not have needed at the time. Although I would have loved to be performing at the Basilica of Saint Mary and also the Saint Paul Cathedral. I did get an invitation to the end of season oratorio banquet; it was held the Monday evening before my Tuesday operation. I would not have been in the right frame of mind for any of this.

But now, almost three months have passed since the diagnosis and over six months since I have been singing; I am thinking, *Music is just too big a part of my life to let it go completely.* And as much as I appreciated having time off from the choir, I start to realize I am really missing it. Also, having cancer makes one a bit selfish, perhaps in a good way. You suddenly realize things can change for you in an instant. No more assuming there are lots of years left to get going on that bucket list, and as far as my free time, I want to start doing more of what I want to do. I've really been letting things go around the house, very unlike me. I call my cleaning service and have them start coming more frequently so I don't have to do quite as much in between. In a pinch, I drop off a load of the kid's laundry at the local dry cleaners. For a period of time, I grow tired of preparing dinner every night; we have Chinese takeout, the local Greek deli, and the Italian restaurant near our house in constant rotation. All this is likely temporary, I realize, but I do find that my priorities have shifted substantially.

I am also reminded, as I am recovering both physically and mentally, of the healing power of music. There are a few moments in my life that I can recall instantly with perfect clarity as though they happened yesterday; the birth of my children comes to mind. But at least for me, many of those amazing, awe-inspiring moments also happen to be during a performance of a choral music masterpiece.

I recall Berlioz Te Deum, Orchestra Hall, January 1, 2000. Despite everyone predicting some sort of doomsday catastrophe, Y2K and all, the performance came off without a hitch. And oh, the ending of that piece! The composer himself exclaimed, "The final movement surpasses all the enormities of which I have been guilty of up to now." It resounded with cymbals crashing, trumpets and coronets blazing, bigger than the *1812 Overture* in my opinion. It perfectly embodied the optimism and the excitement that we all needed to welcome the new millennium. I have had similar almost-out-of-body experiences during Handel's *Dixit Dominus*, Rachmaninoff's *Vespers*, Dvorak's *Stabat Mater*, Rutter's *Requiem*, and many performances of Beethoven's Ninth. Oh, that resounding "Freude"! Every time it sends chills up my spine.

And it's not just the music or the composer that makes this happen. There are also these exquisite moments when our normally reserved, highly professional conductors—I've had two, in twenty years, Dr. George Chu and Dr. Matthew Mehaffey—connect in some otherworldly way with the singers with ethereal results. I'm not the only one who has observed this; after a particularly moving performance three years ago, a fellow oratorio member posted something on Facebook. She writes that part of the motivation for singing comes down to fleeting moments of a very personal relationship between singer and conductor.

"At that instant, through nothing but eye contact, expression, and body language, the conductor will say, 'I will show you everything I am. TRUST me with your soul. I will treasure it and care for it as the precious gift that it is, if only you will follow me.' The performer, in exchange, must give up all emotional control, and trust and simply say, 'My soul is yours for the moment. Lead and I will follow.' It is an exchange of the most deep, intimate, and personal of emotions. It's risky, but when it happens and connects, when it flows through the conduit of beautiful music, it is simply divine . . . a white moment where the body seems to be simply a vessel for something greater."

I read this with intense interest; I knew exactly what she was referring to during Brahms's *Ein Deutsches Requiem*, the day before that Facebook post. Not only is this entire work meltingly beautiful—top three for me, and I have even said (prior to all this!) I want "Wie lieblich" sung at my funeral—but there were several "white moments" in the second, fifth, and the final movements where the connection between conductor, orchestra, and singers felt almost electric. This also happened for me and many others prior to that in an even more emotionally charged piece—Randall Stroope's *Amor de mi Alma*—the last that George Chu conducted before handing over the baton to Matthew Mehaffey. At times, I have found myself trying to sustain a high note with tears welling up or streaming down my face, a difficult feat to say the least. Later, long after the applause has died, this stays with you even when you return to the simple and the mundane, such as going to work the next day, taking call, whittling down the inbox in Epic, even venturing out on Monday evening to attend choir rehearsal when it's twenty degrees below zero.

It turns out, I have truly needed this over the years as a release, an outlet, and a catharsis to the point where in medical school and residency, I would trade call nights and night float shifts just to be able to attend a rehearsal or a performance. All residents submit a "wish list" when creating the yearlong internal medicine residency schedule. My three wishes are for November, March, and May to be ambulatory months instead of inpatient months because these coincide with our regularly scheduled concerts. I am stuck with Christmas pretty much every single year, even later as a faculty member, for this very reason. I think at one point my division director thought I must be Jewish since I seem to be assigned to the inpatient service every December 25. Yes, I find that I am even willing to sacrifice rounding on a holiday in order to continue to experience the beneficial effects of music.

So with this approach in mind, I decide to e-mail my director, Matt Mehaffey. I just want to let him know I'd like to come back for his planning purposes, and I sure as heck hope that he doesn't make me re-audition. Sopranos are the toughest voice part to audition for; there are so many of us, dime a dozen, whereas we always seem to be hurting for tenors and even at times for altos. I mention, "I had somewhat of a health crisis. I needed to have surgery in April, so I was grateful not to have too much on my plate at that time. But now, I really miss it. Singing means the world to me, and I'd like to get back as soon as possible. I'm even interested in the optional Summer Chorus, in addition to the regular season."

He replies, "Heather, this is such great news! Can't wait to see you this summer." I've also copied the chorus manager, Melinda, on this. She writes, "Sorry to hear about the health crisis. So glad you are fine now. Looking forward to seeing you in July." I smile and breathe a sigh of relief. No need to re-audition. I guess I am grandfathered in as I probably should be after . . . twenty years.

So I venture upstairs, and on my bedroom bookshelf is the Schirmer edition of Mendelssohn's *Elijah, An Oratorio*, the vocal score for full chorus, soli, and piano. This is going to be our next performance. I've sung it before; I'm grateful for that. I flip open the cover and look at my penciled-in notes: "May 3rd, Ferguson Hall, Room 85, 9:00 a.m." This must have been the date and location of the dress rehearsal so many years ago. I also see my penciled-in markings across the soprano line, the breath marks, the crescendos and decrescendos, the sit and stand cues.

The very first movement after the overture is for the chorus. The overture builds upon a series of intense chord progressions, which starts tempo moderato, then *poco a poco piu di fuoco* (with gradually increasing animation and fire). It finally reaches a climax, and then *boom*, a sudden and very dramatic slowing of the tempo to andante lento. Then all four vocal parts burst onto the scene in forte:

> Help, Lord!
> Help, Lord!
> Help, Lord!
> Wilt thou quite destroy us?
> Help, Lord.

I read again these lines, thinking *Wow, that is exactly how I felt on the morning of April 5, that Tuesday morning when I got the phone call that the biopsy was positive for cancer. Help, Lord! Will this quite destroy me?*

The entire oratorio moves on to detail the events in the life of the biblical prophet Elijah. There are very dramatic scenes, including the resurrection of a dead youth, the bringing of rain to parched Israel through Elijah's prayers, and the ascension of Elijah on a fiery chariot into heaven. As I continue to flip through the pages of the vocal score, I am struck by how easily the music is coming back to me. I hum the first few bars of "Be not afraid," and it immediately gets stuck in my head for the next several days. I start to sing in the shower, "Blessed are the men who fear Him." I soon realize I am really looking forward to the start of rehearsal, thinking, *This is going to be great.* The music I've sung multiple times—Mozart's *Requiem*, Beethoven's Ninth—is so much more enjoyable than struggling through sight reading every note. And it's actually the opposite of boring or too familiar; it seems as though each and every time, I experience something entirely different, a unique aspect, a new angle on either the vocal expression, the orchestration, or the text.

The most famous chorus from this masterwork is undoubtedly movement 29: "He, watching over Israel." It features a simple yet sweetly beautiful refrain with only a few lines of text.

> He watching over Israel,
> Slumbers not, nor sleeps.
> Shouldst thou walking in grief,
> languish,
> He will quicken thee.

The imagery is very poetic. The above is taken from Psalm 121:4 and Psalm 138:7. Over the coming days, I find myself humming this tune, then dwelling on the text. What comes to mind is the very comforting image of God standing watch over every aspect of our lives—a constant presence. Never for a moment looking away. Never slumbering nor sleeping. Everlasting, eternal, omnipotent, omnipresent.

He is watching, yes, watching over: work, life, relationships, parenting, illness, cancer, anxiety, biopsies, MRI scans, surgery, recovery, medical bills, physical therapy, medications, appointments, follow-up. Despite walking in grief and languishing for the entire month of April, He indeed has quickened my steps once again.

It is such a source of comfort that I continue to let these thoughts dwell, permeate, resonate, bubble up, then down, in, and out continually, just like the triplets that keep coming steadily from the piano line underneath the chorus. Then I start to realize, maybe Mendelssohn as the composer intended those triplets to have exactly this effect. They are the constant, steady, precise, rhythmic notes bubbling up underneath; we as the chorus have the challenge of singing the blissfully expressive line above, but we must execute even eighth notes against the triplet rhythm. It forces you to pay attention to each and every note, both vocally and coming from the piano.

Trip-el-let. Trip-el-let. Trip-el-et. Trip-el-et.

Paul and I often have conversations about music. We both listen to and appreciate a wide variety of artists; our CD collection reflects just about every genre imaginable. But for the most part, I'm a classical choral music singer while he spent years as a self-taught jazz pianist, even playing in cocktail lounges and hotel lobbies in his early twenties—an entirely different approach. Still, we find music is a common ground. I tell him one morning in mid-July about my observations on this Mendelssohn piece. He says, "There is much to connect between theology and music. I would even venture to say, the triplet in music means more than we would ever think from a worldly point of view—it represents the Trinity. Father, Son, and Holy Spirit. This is why the triplet is employed so often by the master composers to convey this concept: the three in one." What a lovely, inspiring thought.

Back in Ted Mann Concert Hall, the first week in August, we are rehearsing the oratorio for the Saturday evening performance. The soloist in the role of Elijah is absolutely amazing—a rising star performing frequently with the Metropolitan Opera. I'm thinking, *How did we ever get this guy?* Worth the price of admission, as they say; the sopranos are all swooning. The orchestra sounds terrific. The strings beautifully mimic the rushing waters. The trumpet blasts accompany the miracles. The horns sound off the famous Elijah chords, announcing his presence. The chorus is coming together very nicely; I am truly amazed at what we have accomplished in a non-auditioned chorale in just eight rehearsals. Even Matt seems impressed, giving us very positive feedback and letting us out early from the Wednesday evening rehearsal.

At the dress rehearsal following along, I am feeling more confident; I am going "off book" quite a bit. I know the notes and the text. I can appreciate the dynamics, the intonation, and everything else. Now, I can simply watch Matt for the cues and rely on him for difficult entrances rather than panic and look down at my score. That's when all the hard work pays off and you can, in a very real sense, merge with the music. And as before, I find, as I am singing, I have those defining moments, especially during "He, watching over Israel" and many other instances in Elijah:

> His mercies on thousands fall . . .
> And, in that still voice, onward
> came the Lord . . .
> Lord, our creator, how excellent thy
> name is . . .

On stage, Saturday evening, August 6, I am having that experience yet again. While connecting with the conductor, the orchestra, and the soloists, I am being transported to another place entirely. In this place, there is only everlasting joy and perfect health; there is no such thing as cancer nor death. Beautiful music flows continually, inimitable harmonies, impeccable tempo, flawless orchestration, superlative chorus, unparalleled dynamics. And of course, every movement—as in "Yet, doth the Lord"—resolves into a perfect C major chord.

This, to me, is the healing power of music. I am fully convinced music is also, in addition to mirth, God's medicine.

And at the end of the oratorio *Elijah*, following the last resounding "Amen," the music ends, the reverb sounds back and dies off, and a standing ovation immediately follows.

I am bathing in it.

EPILOGUE

WHAT THE FUTURE
MAY HOLD

O f course, any person who is going through a serious illness will ask early and often, "Why me? Why is this happening?" I once heard a phrase from Pastor Todd Olson at my church just weeks before this entire ordeal began. Considering trials of various kinds, he said, "It's not 'Why me?' It's 'Why *not* me?'" I tend to agree. Every one of us will have our own health issue someday; it's simply a matter of time. It's the fallen world in which we live in. I reflected on that phrase a lot throughout this entire experience. I have women my age *or younger* in my own clinic who have this same diagnosis. It's stage 3, and it involves much more intense treatment. I also have my panel of patients who have gone through some type of solid organ transplant, are on a complicated and toxic medication regimen, and are always fearful of an infection or a rare malignancy showing up. So while at times it's really challenging to be a physician as patient, it can also give you a perspective that is very helpful.

I have also thought how blessed and how fortunate I am to be on the receiving end of such great care and good outcomes. Sometimes I feel as though I had a "touch" of cancer, but now it's gone, and things are back to normal—sort of like going to the doctor and getting antibiotics and resolving the problem. But just as though one cannot be a "little bit pregnant," I have to recognize and remind myself that this is true of cancer. It will always be a part of me, and the story isn't over yet. And I also know full well the other side of cancer—it doesn't always behave the way we think it will. I know patients who survived years beyond what was predicted, given their stage 4 lung cancer; then I have a young patient succumb to a rare sarcoma in a matter of weeks. I've even seen metastatic breast cancer recurring in women just a few years out from my exact diagnosis, stage, and treatment. So my story is never really over when you look toward the future.

And even if I do end up having a "touch" of cancer, which briefly entered my life, wreaked havoc, and then abruptly left never to return—in a similar fashion to colic in my firstborn child—then again there's the question "Why did it happen in the first place?" At one point, I said to my friend Jodie, "It feels a bit like sausage making, another old cliché. It's as though I am going through some type of meat grinder. It's messy, and I am not really sure what is going to come out the other side, but I hope the end result is something palatable." It's still a bit early to tell, but the insight I have thus far is to make me a better doctor *and* a better patient (as in yes, taking care of oneself once in a while is permissible). To experience the health-care system firsthand. To become a better spouse and a better parent when responding to their needs, their feelings, and everything else that is part of the human experience. Trusting in God, leaning not on my own understanding (Proverbs 3:5–6), but recognizing this is part of a bigger plan. And a huge learning curve for me was giving up control and relying more on the other people in my life— friends, family, church family, colleagues, mentors—and feeling comfortable enough to open up, to share my story.

In the early days, I am tucking Lydia in for the night, sitting on the edge of her bed in between the menagerie of stuffed animals and the pile of books she has been reading. She suddenly asks me, "What if I get breast cancer? And what if it's not stage 1 but stage 4?" After I swallow hard and take a deep breath, I think, *Where is she getting this stuff?* I guess children overhear more of the conversations around this house than I think they do. Then I remember, her friend Ella also shared the story about her grandfather having stage 4 pancreatic cancer. Too much for young children to have to contemplate cancer staging, but there it is; I can't take it back.

"Well," I say, not really sure how to answer. "Just to be certain, you will have X-rays to look for this years ahead of time, even younger than me." By my own calculation and also the recommendation of the genetic counselor, probably around age thirty-four.

"You mean an MRI? I don't want to have an MRI!" she says.

Whoa. Again, those big ears hearing me describe how loud and confining the machine felt. "Well, yes, probably an MRI. Or by then, some newfangled high-tech total body scan that can evaluate for any type of cancer anywhere in the body!"

This sounds a bit like science fiction. Both of my kids can relate; in recent years, they've been into the sci-fi series *Doctor Who* to the point that Sam dressed up as the Eleventh Doctor for Halloween, complete with pompadour hair, dark-red bow tie, tan jacket, sonic screwdriver—perfection. Also, they have decided to call our never-ending rotation of full-time nannies, summer nannies, after-school nannies "the doctors." It's a perfect analogy. On the show, at about the end of every third season, there is a "regeneration, renewal, change of appearance," and lo and behold, a new doctor appears who is there to protect innocent people from harm and restore order in the universe, which is definitely how I view my nannies.

But when I talk about high-tech imaging and other possibilities, it's not just sci-fi to me. It's very real and awe-inspiring to think where this field will be in ten to fifteen years. I've shared this perspective with my medical students a lot. When I was an intern in 1998, left and right I was admitting patients with pneumocystis pneumonia, crypto meningitis, and other late-stage complications of HIV. Now, HIV is a chronic disease with a near-normal life expectancy, and crypto meningitis is a rare diagnosis for morning report or M&M. When I was a brand-new attending on service in 2002, the resident was presenting a patient who was just started on Gleevec for chronic myelogenous leukemia. "What the heck is Gleevec?" I ask. Thank God I'm at a teaching hospital; we can ask each other questions. It turns out the five-year survival for people with CML doubled from around 30 percent to 60 percent with the approval of this tyrosine kinase inhibitor drug in 2001. I'm also thinking about hepatitis C; it used to be the scourge of our hemophiliacs prior to routine screening of the blood supply and an unfortunate long-term consequence of risky lifestyle choices and the most common indication for liver transplantation. Now, a simple screening blood test followed by popping a pill once a day for twelve weeks—Harvoni—and the patient doesn't have to feel like death warmed over on interferon.

So looking ahead, in terms of breast cancer, I believe there are endless possibilities in terms of earlier diagnosis, better treatment, management. I even shared this with Lydia that evening before bed. First, I responded to her feelings, validating her fears, sharing how I had been coping myself—music, writing, and exercise. I then reassured her that there is no hereditary component to my diagnosis, best we can tell. And I tried to end on a positive note, mentioning how advances in the field will benefit future patients.

As far as me, personally, looking toward the future, I have additional goals and plans moving forward. I've gotten back to running and golf. I have rejoined the Oratorio Society for all of next season; the repertoire chosen by Matthew Mehaffey is outstanding, including next summer, Brahms's *Ein Deutsches Requiem*. An all-time favorite of mine! *Ewige freude.*

I've also decided that, given how much I seem to enjoy writing, I really need to finish those two (okay, *four*) half-written manuscripts that are on my desktop, waiting to be submitted to an academic journal, on topics such as direct observation in resident clinic, a novel interprofessional curriculum, and even mentorship in academic medicine. Although looking at the survey results from our newly implemented mentoring program, I start thinking, *We asked all the wrong questions here. I don't see anything about someone covering your small group so you can have surgery.* I'm also writing a case report of axillary web syndrome with Todd Tuttle and Linda Koehler—yes, my own, complete with photos. This is a lot of potential publications! I sincerely hope, however, that I will not need to be struck by a second cancer just so I can get another two weeks off work to fully devote to the writing process. Maybe I can just ask for a sabbatical instead?

And for once, my venturing out and presenting at an academic meeting pays off even if it is mere days after having surgery. Yes, thinking back to Baltimore. Shortly thereafter, I am sitting at a committee meeting for medical school course directors when our new associate dean, Dr. Bob Englander, stops by to pay a visit. He mentions how we need to incorporate more active learning into our curriculum. He even goes on to describe a new grant program that he is willing to support our time—10 percent of our salary—for faculty to innovate and try something new. All the while, I'm listening with intense interest, thinking, *This might be exactly what I need to further along the online modules and other projects.* After the meeting, I e-mail him, giving a brief summary of our work, mentioning that we just presented at Johns Hopkins in May. I even include a link to our abstract on the MedBiquitous website. Dr. Englander replies less than five minutes later: "Dear Heather, I would be delighted to meet. I have to admit I had already heard of your work and was hoping you would be excited about the invitation this morning. Let's try to have lunch." Wow, now that was a door opening.

And many months later, while at AAMC in Atlanta, I just happen to bump into a colleague from Louisville whom I also met at this Baltimore meeting, Dr. Tao Le. We are standing in the refreshment area when he happens to mention he is developing an online, portable, fully customizable curriculum for the second year of medical school, and the first organ system is *hematology*. We exchange cards and meet later for lunch. To this day, our collaboration on a national curriculum using evidence-based teaching methods continues.

Also, when I contemplate the future, another favorite passage from the Old Testament Bible comes to mind: Proverbs 31:10–31.

The verses are an acrostic poem, each verse beginning with the successive letters of the Hebrew alphabet. It has often been called "The Ideal Woman" or "The Wife of Noble Character."

While reading that entire list can be a bit intimidating, I appreciate several of the references:

26   She opens her mouth with wisdom,
      and the teaching of kindness is on her tongue.

27   She looks well to the ways of her household
      and does not eat the bread of idleness.

28   Her children rise up and call her blessed. (NASB)

And my personal favorite:

25   Strength and dignity are her clothing,
      and she laughs at the days to come. (NASB)

I found many instances of humor in this entire endeavor; although early on, it was harder to laugh when I just wanted to cry. As things moved forward, clearing several hurdles, with a few more reassurances, more good test results, then it became easier. And I sincerely hope, even though medicine is at times a very serious business, that perhaps health-care professionals who are reading this can appreciate that having a sense of humor is a very worthwhile approach. Laughter is, as they say, the very best medicine.

So to summarize, I am now to the point where I feel I could finally do just that—*laugh at the days to come.*

Stand

Song by Blues Traveler

The answers are getting harder and harder

And there ain't no way to bargain or to barter

But if you've got the angst, or the ardor—

You might faint from the fight, but you're gonna find it

For every challenge could have paradise behind it

And if you accept what you have lost, and you stand tall,

You might just get it back,

And you can get it all.

About the Author

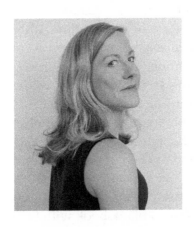

Dr. Heather Thompson Buum is an assistant professor at the University of Minnesota in the Division of General Internal Medicine. She graduated from Hamline University in 1993 with a BA in biology, then went on to complete both medical school and residency at the University of Minnesota. She joined the faculty in 2002 and devotes half her time to patient care, practicing both outpatient primary care and inpatient hospital medicine. The remaining time, she spends in various teaching and administrative roles. She formerly served as an associate program director for the internal medicine residency and now is a course director for Human Health and Disease and a small group facilitator for Essentials of Clinical Medicine in the medical school. Dr. Thompson has won numerous awards for both teaching and patient care, including Outstanding Medical School Teacher in 2016, the Department of Medicine Clinical Excellence Award in 2013, and *Minnesota Monthly*'s Top Doctors for Women in 2013 and 2011. She is a member of the Society for General Internal Medicine and a fellow in the American College of Physicians. Her outside interests include choral music, performing with the Oratorio Society of Minnesota for over twenty years. She also enjoys cooking, running, and an occasional round of golf. She lives with her husband and two children in St. Paul.

ACKNOWLEDGMENTS

This book began as a suggestion from my astute friend Amanda. Early on, I had been telling her story after story regarding this new diagnosis. Some of them were frightening, many of them heartwarming, several quite ironic, and a few downright humorous. She says to me, driving in the car one day, "You really should be writing all of this down. As you move on and things seem a little more distant, you want to be able to remember everything that happened." I thought, *What a good idea.* And once the tamoxifen and/or chemo turns my brain into mush, well, the details might get lost.

During this time, I also had a care package sent to me in the mail, including a journal, a lovely lined blank book with blue and purple flowers on the cover. I thought, *Huh, I have not done any journaling since college.* I tried jotting down a few notes with pen and paper, but after spending over a decade typing my own progress notes into the electronic medical record, I came to realize I am a lightning-fast typist. Makes sense, wouldn't it? I completed a typing class in high school back when it was *called* typing; it's a reinforceable skill. My speed improves year after year. So instead, I open Google Docs on my Google Drive, type "Chapter 1," and the rest, as they say, is history. And as opposed to writing a grant proposal or drafting a manuscript for an academic journal, this one was easy for me. Page after page simply flowed; after each new experience, I would think, *Well, that's got to be another chapter in the book.*

It was just, as they say, cheaper than therapy. Nearing the end of my project, I had to decide if this remained on my Google Drive, visible only to me, as tangible evidence of my own coping skills, or if somehow others might benefit from reading it. I'm not the type who wants to draw attention to myself; this was truly way out of my comfort zone. But I realized that even if one person resonates with the story or finds a bit of encouragement or even just enjoys a good laugh, well then, it is probably worth it. The ultimate goal of my writing was to share a story so that others may benefit, offering hope, encouragement, or maybe just a candid glimpse into the world of medicine and what to expect when entering our health-care system—good, bad, or otherwise.

Of course, I simply must thank my family and friends who supported me along the way in this endeavor, but time and space do not permit me to list them all here. I have my own mini editorial staff at the Buum house: Sam and Lydia, who have read entire chapters and given me feedback, and Paul, who helped me settle on a title and design the cover art. I want to thank Charlie Moldow as the first person to read my book when it was all of eighteen chapters and gave me the encouragement to keep writing. And I credit my mom, Vicki, for instilling in me at a very young age the love of reading. Because as author and oncologist Siddhartha Mukherjee said, "The cardinal rule of learning to write is learning to read first."

More importantly, this work is dedicated to the patients, nurses, staff, doctors, fellows, residents, and medical students at the University of Minnesota. Even prior to this, I would have said, *you* are the reason I am still here despite having to adjust to a new clinic building, navigate potential health-system mergers, endure occasional bad press from the local newspaper, constantly adapt to new leadership, struggle through promotion and tenure tracks, and all the other strife that seems to be a part of academic medicine. Now, well, my heartfelt appreciation has risen to a whole new level. Those who trained me as a doctor are now taking care of me as a patient. It's the ultimate full circle and illustrates the connectedness of us all.

Coming Soon:
With Mirth and Laughter

With mirth and laughter let old wrinkles come.
And let my liver heat with wine
than my heart cool with mortifying groans.
—William Shakespeare, Merchant of Venice

A continuation of the story, *With Mirth and Laughter: Finding Joy in Medicine after Cancer*, is Dr. Heather Thompson Buum's second book. It now moves beyond the early days of breast cancer treatment, including surgery, medication, and physical therapy, and further describes how a cancer diagnosis affects her friendships, family dynamics, and teaching and mentoring roles. More importantly, it continues to change her practice style and her view of what it means to provide patient-centered care. This book includes story after story of patient interactions, some ironic, many humorous, but all poignant and compelling; they serve to illustrate how being in one role ultimately benefits the other.

Dr. Thompson also chronicles how becoming a patient informs her role as a medical educator, changing her approach in how she teaches and trains future physicians. Those in academic medicine or in a teaching role of any kind can relate. Cancer survivors, as well as health-care providers, will appreciate the observations and shift in perspective as she moves from doctor as patient to patient as doctor. All the while, Dr. Thompson keeps her keen sense of humor, sharing many amusing stories about primary care, academic medicine, and even the somewhat harrowing process of becoming a writer.

You can read more about the book *With Mirth and Laughter* at *www.doctor-heather.com*. It will be available online at Barnes and Noble and Amazon and in the Coffman Union Bookstore at the University of Minnesota.